MENDING THE TORN FABRIC

For Those Who Grieve and Those Who Want To Help Them

Sarah Brabant, Ph.D., C.C.S.
University of Southwestern Louisiana

Death, Value and Meaning Series
Series Editor: John D. Morgan

Baywood Publishing Company, Inc.
AMITYVILLE, NEW YORK

Library of Congress Catalog Number: 96-14887
ISBN: 0-89503-141-8 (cloth : alk. paper)

Library of Congress Cataloging-in-Publication Data

Brabant, Sarah.
   Mending the torn fabric : for those who grieve and those who want
to help them / Sarah Brabant.
      p. cm. — (Death, value and meaning series)
   Includes bibliographical references and index.
   ISBN 0-89503-141-8 (cloth : alk. paper)
   1. Bereavement- -Psychological aspects. 2. Grief. I. Title.
II. Series.
BF575.G7B72   1996
155.9'37- -dc20
                                                              96-14887
                                                                   CIP

ACKNOWLEDGMENTS

I first began to use the analogy of a torn fabric in my work with bereaved persons in the late 1980s. It seemed to be an effective tool, and I shared this with Elizabeth Clark on a plane returning from Spain after a meeting of the International Sociological Association. She invited me to write an article about the analogy for a new journal she planned to edit [1]. Subsequently she and two other clinical sociologists, Julia Mayo and Beverley Cuthbertson-Johnson, encouraged me to develop the analogy still further.

Several persons who know grief all too well, Nancy Goodwin, Cheryl and Bill Guidry, Sally McKissack, and "D," were gracious enough to read an early draft of this book. Their comments were insightful and encouraging. Sister Elizabeth Loomis, S.H.C.J., at that time on the staff of a near-by retreat center, read an early draft and was also encouraging. C. Eddie Palmer, a clinical sociologist, and Pat Andrus, a grief counselor, provided critical commentary on a later version. My husband and colleague, Wilmer MacNair, read numerous drafts and often served as a sounding board for me. Diane Moore offered much needed editorial assistance. Several professionals, Catherine Cox, a massage therapist, and physicians, W. A. Bernard, Enoch Callaway, and Enoch Brabant, critiqued sections pertinent to their fields. In the final phase, John D. Morgan and two anonymous reviewers provided further guidance. I am indebted to all of these persons. I also want to thank my sister-in-law, Dorothy Callaway, for her many years of support and encouragement.

Words are inadequate to express my appreciation to the owner of the dream. Perhaps allowing me to share your precious gift will give hope to those who continue to yearn for some sign. Your story and the stories of others are the heart of this book.[1] It is to you and to all of the other bereaved men, women, and children who have permitted me to see your frayed and ragged fabrics, to watch your courageous attempts (both the failures and the successes) to mend your tears, and to behold the indescribably beautiful tapestries that unfold as mending takes place that I dedicate this book.

REFERENCE

1. S. Brabant, Mending the Torn Fabric: An Analogy for Grief Counseling, *Illness, Crisis, and Loss* 1:1 pp. 49-53, 1991.

---

[1] Many of the stories are presented just as they were told to me. Some, however, have been slightly altered to protect anonymity.

CONTENTS

Chapter 1

THE TORN FABRIC

The meeting of Compassionate Friends, a support group for bereaved parents, was over. The guest speaker and most of the parents had left. I was helping with the clean-up when one of the remaining parents walked over to me. "I'm so tired of people coming here and telling me how I feel," she said angrily. "I know I'm in pain, but I can't get a handle on it. I know what grief feels like; I don't know what it looks like." I listened as she poured out her frustration. After a few minutes, she thanked me for listening, and went on her way. As I gathered up my things and went out to get in my car, I kept thinking about what she had said. "I know what grief feels like; I don't know what it looks like."

This woman's child had died and she was in enormous pain. She knew the source of her pain. She knew what her pain felt like. She wanted to know what her pain looked like. Perhaps if she could somehow see the pain, she could "get a handle" on it. As I mulled her words over and over in my mind, I pictured a torn fabric, badly in need of mending. I saw a person bending over this torn fabric trying to sew the edges of the tear together. No matter how this person tried to mend the tear, the rip tore open again and again and I thought, that is what the terrible pain of grief looks like. It is a tear that keeps tearing no matter how hard you try to mend it. What does a person do when that happens? Do you just live with this enormous tear in your fabric or do you keep searching until you find the right needles and threads to mend it? Can such a badly torn fabric ever be mended?

As a support person for a Compassionate Friends chapter for over ten years, I have attended too many meetings and listened to too many bereaved parents not to know the answer. You keep working on your mending and, sooner or later, you find the right needles and threads. It takes time, sometimes a long time, and it takes work, sometimes a great deal of work, but even the most torn fabric can be mended. It will never be the same as it once was, but there will come a time when the fabric's owner can once again focus on the fabric itself rather than just on mending it.

This does not just happen as a matter of course. Mending is work and it takes time and patience. Even before we can begin to look for the right needles and threads, we have to acknowledge that there is a break, a tear,[1] in our fabric. Then we have to become familiar with the tear. We have to comprehend the size of it, its outline, and where it is in our fabric. Is it only a small tear, a medium size tear, or one almost as big as the fabric itself? Is it a round hole or a jagged rip? Is it in a corner of our fabric or in the center? And we have to know what kind of fabric we are working with. Not all tears are the same; not all fabrics are the same. We may need to use different needles and threads at different times in the mending process. We may need to learn new stitches. That is what this book is all about. It is about tears and needles and threads and stitches. This book is about mending a torn fabric.

Think of your life, your very being, as a piece of fabric. When you were born you were given this piece of fabric. No one else has ever been given this particular piece of fabric before. It is your fabric and it is unique. The material may be similar to that of others; it may be very different. Some people, for example, get a piece of Irish linen. This kind of material is sturdy and is not easily torn. Most stains are easily removed with laundry detergent; even the worst stain can usually be removed with bleach. If the fabric is torn, just about any needle can be used for mending

---

[1] The word "tear" has two distinctly different meanings: 1) a hole or flaw made by tearing; and 2) a drop of clear saline secreted from the eye. To avoid confusion, "tear" or "tears" will always refer to a torn place or a rip in a piece of fabric and never to the liquid that flows from a person's eyes when he or she is crying.

as long as the needle is strong enough and sharp enough to pierce the fabric. Others, however, may be given a piece of Swiss batiste. This delicate material is beautiful, shimmering with light as you finger it. But you have to be very careful with this kind of cloth. Most stain removers will damage the material and only very small, sharp needles can be used. A large needle will leave a hole; a dull one will rip into the fabric, leaving pulled threads and sometimes even a ragged tear.

There are so many different kinds of materials in the world. There are the heavy cottons, the ginghams, the various kinds of woolens, the silks; there is khaki, denim, and burlap. Even when materials are the same, there are differences in weaves and dyes. Brothers and sisters who share the same biological parents have different fabrics, because it makes a difference whether a piece of fabric is cut at the beginning of the bolt, or the middle, or the end. Were you the oldest child in your family, the youngest child, the only child? Even if you are an identical twin, you or your twin is the oldest; the other is the youngest. Your fabric is unique. It always has been. It always will be.

Time affects all fabrics. Some people use their fabrics every day until the cloth is worn in places from so much use. Others choose to do nothing with their material, storing it away in a closet for some future use. Even so, the cloth does not stay the same. It may yellow with age and even become weakened in places so that when it is used, it tears more readily. Some persons choose to decorate their fabric, painting designs upon it or embroidering it. Sometimes the design is so beautiful that it becomes a cherished keepsake for others, perhaps many others. Sometimes a design does not turn out too well. The owner may decide to live with it, paint over it, or rip it out and begin a new design.

As we move through life, we are often careless with our fabric. We lay it down somewhere or leave it unattended and it becomes soiled (e.g., we become bored or we lose muscle tone). Perhaps another person spills something on our fabric (e.g., gossip damages our reputation). These stains often can be removed if we find the right cleanser; sometimes the stain cannot be removed no matter what we do. We may even tear our fabric trying to get the stain out. At other times we may notice a little tear in our fabric and wonder how it happened. We may decide to ignore it since it is so little, or we may mend it with a quick stitch or two. Sometimes, however, our fabric becomes so torn that we cannot ignore the tear or hastily repair it. A particular tear may be so huge that it is difficult to even see the fabric. We wonder if such a tear can ever be mended. Maybe the tear is so large that the fabric is useless forevermore.

Through the years I have listened to the stories of many grieving people. They have shared with me some tears in their fabrics that were so big and so jagged that the fabric appeared irreparable. And I have watched as these courageous men, women, and children began the task of mending their torn fabrics. It often takes a long time and sometimes the stitches they take seem to do more damage than good. I have watched them try one stitch and then another. I have seen newly-stitched tears rip open again. I have watched as the person began to mend the tear once more and, this time, found a thread that could hold the ragged edges together. I have come to believe that no fabric is beyond mending. With enough time and enough work, even the most terrible tear can be mended to the point that the material can once again be vibrant.

There are many different kinds of tears and they vary in size. There are also many different kinds of needles and threads. Before talking about different kinds of tears, needles, and threads, however, there are four words that are important for us to define. These words are *bereavement, grief, grief work,* and *mourning.* These words do not mean the same thing, and unfortunately two of these words, *grief work* and *mourning,* are often confused with each other. It would be nice if there were some universal consensus about the definition of these words, but it is not essential. What is important is to recognize that there are four very different dimensions in the grieving process, and that you and I use the same word to describe each of these dimensions.

The first word is *bereavement.* A bereavement is a loss. It can be any loss. Bereavement simply means that something you once had is no longer yours. Have you ever lost your keys? This is a bereavement. Most of the time this is not a very important bereavement or loss because you probably had a duplicate key at home or you asked a locksmith to make a new key for you. But it was a loss and demanded your attention if only for a little time. These kinds of losses are inconvenient losses. They are a nuisance, but they are easily taken care of. Other losses are not so easy to take care of. We may lose our job or find out that a person we thought was a friend was talking about us behind our back. We may eventually find a new job or make new friends, but until we do there is a great emptiness in our life. And even when we have been in our new job for a time or become comfortable around our new friends, we may feel pain when we remember the way things were.

Sometimes a bereavement or loss is so enormous that life seems to come to a standstill. From that moment on, one's life is divided into before the loss and after the loss. For a parent, a child's death is this kind of bereavement. Never, never, never can that child be replaced. There may be other children to come, but that unique child is no longer physically present and that child's presence cannot be duplicated. A bereavement or loss, then, is a tear in our fabric. It can be a little tear, hardly noticeable. It can be a medium size tear that demands attention, but only for a time. It can be a tear so devastating that the bereaved person wonders if his or her fabric can ever be mended.

Grief is the human response to loss. It is the pain a person feels when someone or something that was important in his or her life is no longer present. Grief can be momentary or it can last a long time. It can be so temporary that we quickly forget it. It can be so overwhelming that it is difficult to breathe and we wonder if we will physically survive our loss, much less emotionally survive it. What is important to remember is that there can be a bereavement or loss and little or no pain. If there is pain, however, there is always a loss. If the pain is great, the loss is large. This is an important axiom to keep in mind and we will return to it in later chapters. For now, just remember that there can be a loss with no pain, but if there is pain, there is always a tear in your fabric.

Grief work is the work that must be done to move through the pain that we experience because of a loss. The word "through" is important. You cannot just go around the pain or under the pain or over the pain; the only way to go is through the pain. Until you do this, the pain will surround you and if it is intense enough, the pain will control your life. When you go through the pain, the pain becomes a part of you. Thus, there is nowhere to go with pain but through it. You may never be free of the pain, but you can learn to live with it. It will cease to control your life. Grief work, then, is the necessary mending that has to be done in order to move through the pain. Work is a good term, for it reminds us that there is something we have to do in order to move through the pain. The pain will not just go away. A torn fabric will not just mend by itself.

Finally there is the word *mourning*. Some people use this word when they are talking about grief work. We will use it to mean certain kinds of grief work (i.e., grief work that is approved by the members of any particular society). In other words, mourning is how our cultural background (nationality, ethnicity, religion) teaches us how we should respond, and how we think others will expect us to respond to our losses. We can recognize mourning when we use or hear phrases such as "I think (or others think) that I should feel a certain way" or "I think (or others think) I ought to do certain things." With respect to grief work, there is often a particular way of behaving that is considered appropriate by ourselves or others and to behave differently is to risk disapproval. Our cultural background, however, provides more than just ways of responding to loss. It also tells us how important our loss is, whether we have a right to hurt, and if so, how much and for how long.

Mourning, then, is how a culture defines the tear in our fabric. Is the tear a big one or only a small one? Mourning is how our culture tells us we should feel about our tears and how, or even if, we can express our pain. Mourning is how our culture defines mending for us. What is and what is not acceptable?

Mourning definitions and rules may be very helpful; they may also keep us from moving through the grieving process. Only you know how big the tear is in your fabric because only you know how much you hurt. Only you can do the mending. It is very important, however, to recognize mourning. What others think about bereavement, grief, and grief work or what we have learned to think about bereavement, grief, and grief work can prevent us from getting our mending done. It can even prevent us from beginning our mending.

We will talk about some of the barriers that can block us from our mending and how to get around these blocks in more detail. Before continuing on to the next chapter, however, it might help to repeat the following affirmations several times.

My fabric is unique.

If I am hurting, there is a tear in my fabric.

Since only I know how much I hurt, only I know how big the tear is.

My fabric can be mended.

Chapter 2

PLACES TO MEND

About twenty-five years ago a young physician who worked with dying patients was asked to write a book about dying and death. Today this would not seem so strange, but back in the 1960s dying and death were taboo topics for many people. Dying persons in hospitals were often moved to rooms at the far end of the hall, and when they died their body was bundled up and hurriedly sent to a morgue as though the person had done something so terrible in dying that it must be kept secret. This courageous physician dared to call this kind of treatment of dying persons shameful. She argued that dying persons should be respected because they have a right to this respect and also because they have much to teach the living. She accepted the challenge to write a book and today people all over the world recognize the name, Elisabeth Kübler-Ross, and many have read her book, *On Death and Dying* [1]. Indeed, many still refer to this book as *the* book on death and dying.

Elisabeth Kübler-Ross never intended for her book to become *the* book on death and dying. In the preface, she wrote:

> I am simply telling the stories of my patients who shared their agonies, their expectations, and their frustrations with us. It is hoped that it will encourage others not to shy away from the "hopelessly" sick but to get closer to them, as they can help them much during their final hours [1, preface].

Unfortunately, we live in a "cookbook society." We want step-by-step directions on how to do things, and since few people at that time had any idea of what a dying person was going through, her

9

book became the guideline for what to expect. Not too much was known about grieving either, so the book became the guideline for the grieving process as well. Even today, many people continue to describe the grief process as five stages: denial, bargaining, anger, depression, and acceptance. According to them, it is quite simple. You have a loss and then you move through each of the stages and when you have completed the first four stages, you reach acceptance. That is all there is to it. You are now through with your grief.

Well, it is not that simple. And Elisabeth Kübler-Ross never said it was that simple. I often wonder if either the people who claim the grief process is that simple or those who criticize her book as being too simplistic have ever really read it. It is a wonderful book and she did just exactly what she said she was going to do. She listened to her patients and she shared their stories with those who read her book. She was allowing others to hear those stories, not trying to establish a format of predictable behavior. Her use of the word "stage," however, may have inadvertently encouraged people who were looking for some direction to think of the dying and/or grieving process as a predictable sequence of steps.

Words are more than meaning; they point us in one direction or another. Stop and think for a moment what the word "stage" means. I think of steps that go higher and higher and you have to climb the first one before you can reach the next one. Grade levels in school are an example of stages. You have to complete first grade in order to go to second grade. If you do not complete first grade, it means you have failed and that is a terrible thing to do. But what about being promoted to second and then being sent back to first? That is even worse than failing. It means you have slipped and that is something only weak people do. If you do not slip, however, but keep climbing higher and higher, you reach the final stage—graduation—and that is wonderful. Regression is shameful; graduation is cause for celebration.

Because the word "stage" makes us think in terms of ordered steps and failing and succeeding, I prefer to use the word "place." A place is simply a location in which we find ourself at any given point in time. One place is not necessarily better or worse or higher or lower than another place. A place is simply a space that can be occupied at any given time. Elisabeth Kübler-Ross said that the dying person may move from one place (stage) to another and back again any number of times. This is also true for grieving persons. An individual may move from one place to another only to return again to an earlier place. He or she may move from place to place rapidly or remain in one place for a long period of time. Wherever you are at any given time is where you are. One place is neither higher nor lower than another. Each place is different. It does help, however, to be able to recognize where you are, or as one bereaved woman told me, it helps at least to know where you have been.

To describe all of the possible places a bereaved person might enter would be a book in and of itself. There are, however, several places that most bereaved persons enter at one time or another. One place all bereaved persons probably enter at some time is the place of denial. Note that I said "one place," not "first place." We are not talking about stages; we are talking about places. You may have already been in this place if your fabric is torn; you may have entered and exited it a number of times. You may enter it again. Actually, denial is not a single place. There are several places of denial. They are similar, but each is a little different.

DENIAL

Sometimes the tear in a fabric is so sudden that the person may not realize that there really is a tear. Denial does not mean that the person is mentally slow or emotionally weak. It takes time to fully comprehend that a tear has occurred. A person thinks, "Maybe there really isn't a tear. I just thought there was. Tomorrow I will see that my fabric is really unchanged." But then tomorrow comes, and the tear is still there. He or she did not just dream the phone call or the trip to the emergency room. It is true. His or her loved one is dead. His or her fabric is torn.

Sometimes it takes weeks or months, sometimes even years, to fully comprehend that a loved one has died. This often happens when death is sudden and unexpected. Parents whose children were killed have told me that it took six months or more to fully comprehend that their child was really dead, and that the pain was even more intense then than it was right after the death. They often add, "I guess I was just in denial." And they say this to me as though they are confessing some terrible sin for which they are ashamed. "How," they ask me, "could I deny my own child's death?" It is important to remember that being in a place of denial has nothing to do with strength or weakness. When something terrible happens, when a person's fabric is so terribly ripped, the body shuts down, preventing the mind from fully comprehending what has happened. This is not a sign of weakness; it is a natural protection.

Bereaved persons often share with me that they perceive their earlier denial as some sort of weakness on their part or a betrayal of the person they loved. I ask them if they have noticed any recent changes with respect to taste, or preference of some kind. One man thought about this question for a moment or two and then said that he had hated squash all his life and would always refuse to eat it. During the first year following his son's death, however, he had eaten whatever was placed in front of him, even squash. He did not care what he ate. He really did not care if he ate. Recently, however, he refused to eat squash because of his distaste for that food.

Others have commented on temperature. One woman told me that following her daughter's death she was cold all of the time, regardless of what the thermometer said. It was almost a shock to her when she realized one day that she was too warm. Another woman said that for months after her husband's death she put on whatever was at hand. Mixing or matching colors was unimportant. One day she happened to catch a glimpse of herself in a mirror and was startled at how badly her blouse clashed with her skirt. A sudden loss, then, affects the physical body. As the body slowly recovers from the terrible shock of loss, so does the mind. You may become more aware of taste or temperature or colors. Your emotional pain may also seem to intensify.

It is very similar to cutting your finger. At first you cannot believe that you let the knife slip. Surely you did not really cut yourself. You then realize that your finger is cut, but it seems to be only a small cut. Then you begin to notice blood. You may try to stop the bleeding for a time. Then you decide your finger is bleeding too profusely. You need help. Eventually you go to the emergency room or clinic and get stitches. It may be later that night or even the next day before you really become aware of the pain. This slow awakening to the magnitude of a physical injury is a natural process that protects the mind from too much pain too soon. Unfortunately in our culture, this built-in protection gets twisted into some sort of notion of being weak, especially with respect to grief.

This physical, mental, and emotional shutdown following a death is common when the death is sudden. It may also occur when death is anticipated but not expected to happen immediately. Following the death of his partner from AIDS, one man kept telling me over and over, "I knew he was going to die, but he wasn't supposed to die this soon." For several days following the death, he would hold a lighted cigarette between his fingers, oblivious of how far it had burned down. At one point he apparently did burn his finger, but seemed unaware of any discomfort. A friend, noticing the burn, took care of it for him.

Denial associated with the shock of unexpectedly losing an important person, then, can follow any death and can be relatively short-term or long-lasting. Emerging from this place of denial, especially if you have been in it for weeks or months, can be frightening. The sudden intensified pain may seem overwhelming. It may help to remember that, just as with a cut finger, the awareness of pain is a sign of healing, not weakness or failure.

A bereaved person may also move into a place of denial following an expected, even yearned for, death. Entry into this place of denial, however, is different from the one just described. At the end of a long illness, death may be welcomed by both the person who is dying, as well as the person who will be left behind. No one wants to see a loved one suffer. Not all thoughts, however, are on the beloved. Taking care of a dying person is an arduous task. A person who is exhausted from staying up all night may pray for release. No one can tell you when the actual death will occur; you wonder how many more nights you can go with little or no sleep. Caregivers often share with me that they do not know how much more they can take, physically or emotionally. Thus, a person may long for death because of compassion for the person in pain. He or she may also long for death as an end to caretaking. The first reason is generally accepted in our society. The second reason often causes people problems, because it is often defined as self-centered. Both reasons, however, are very human.

One man told me that all he felt the day after his partner died was relief that it was over. He was not sad; he was not angry; he was just relieved. A week later he told me that he must have been in denial following the death and that he just felt terrible about feeling relieved, and even more terrible that it had taken him over a week to realize that the person he loved more than anyone else he had ever known was gone forever. Although he never denied his loved one's death, he had denied the magnitude of his loss. Because of this, he felt he had somehow betrayed their relationship. Again, a bereaved person has defined the place of denial as an indication of personal weakness.

The defining characteristic of denial may make this a particularly frightening place for many persons. By definition, we cannot know when we are in denial because if we did know then we would not be in denial. Denial, then, is the only place we can never recognize we are in at the time we are in it. We can only recognize it after we have exited. For many people, even the thought of not knowing where he or she is at any given moment can be terrifying. Such thoughts are often equated with being crazy, a fear many bereaved persons have regardless of the place they are in at that moment.

It may be helpful for you to think of denial as a place of resting before the mending begins. If you really grasped immediately how ragged your fabric was, you might be tempted to throw it away, or you might try to mend it too hastily and cause even greater damage to your material. However, if you sit for a time and let the tear slowly enter your consciousness, if you allow yourself time to become aware of the magnitude of the tear, you will be stronger and better able to begin the work of mending.

Think of entering a room with a basket filled with mending to be done. You are tired. You could try to get your mending done, but you probably will do a poor job and have much of it to do again. Just sitting in a chair, doing nothing, may be the best thing you can do. The torn cloth will be there when you once again focus on it, and you will be better prepared to attend to it.

The places of denial allow our body and mind a needed respite, for in these places our fabric is hidden or at least partially hidden from us. The places of denial are gifts. No one enters denial willingly. We do not even know we have been there until we exit. We do not exit until our body and mind are able to withstand the rigors of places to come.

It is important to remember that denial is not a single place that once exited is never re-entered. Indeed not. You may first deny that your fabric is really torn, then realize that it is. You may still deny that the tear is such a large one, then recognize that it is. You may think that you can mend it quickly, and finally comprehend that it is going to take a long time to repair. You have been moving in and out of places of denial, each similar to the other and yet each a little different. Each time you enter one of these places, you enter a new resting place in your mending process. Each time you exit one of these resting places, you emerge a little more knowledgeable about the state of your fabric, and are better able to begin the next mending task before you. You needed this place of rest before really seeing the enormity of the tear, or before realizing that you need to find new needles or a different kind of thread. You may even ultimately need this place of rest before you decide that the time has come to set your mending basket aside and once more begin to paint or embroider your fabric. If you are just exiting a place of denial, your pain may seem more intense than before. Remember that you would not have exited the place of denial if you were not ready to continue on your journey through this pain. Intensified pain is not a sign of weakness or failure; it is a sign of strength and healing.

There is a place that is often confused with denial. I have had people ask me if I thought they were in denial. Someone has died and they feel little or no pain. The fact that they ask indicates they are not denying a tear. It is, of course, possible that they are blocking the pain. There is also the possibility that they have a tear that has already been mended. They mended the tear before the person died. This is called *anticipatory grieving*. When an illness is prolonged over years, and especially when there has been mental deterioration, the person you knew and loved died long before the actual physical death. You may have continued to visit him or her. Perhaps you were the primary caregiver. You cared for a person who was alive, but the person you knew and loved was dead. When this happens, your grief work may have begun and even been completed before the physical death occurs.

Following one of my workshops, I received a letter from a woman thanking me for explaining anticipatory grief. Her father lived in a distant city, but she visited him often. They had a close relationship, and she looked forward to their times together. After his stroke, however, this changed. He was in a coma for almost a year. She continued her visits, but did so out of duty. She dreaded the long drive twice a month. On her way home she would weep for the father she had known and lost. When her father died, however, she felt only relief. She was ashamed of what she defined as insensitivity and hoped that she might be in denial. At the workshop she realized that she had grieved the loss of her father throughout the year before he actually died.

ANGER

Denial is only one of the places bereaved persons commonly enter. Another place in which many people spend time following a loss is the place of anger. You may be angry at the tear itself, or angry at the person whose death caused the tear. You may be angry at physicians, lawyers, office workers; you may be angry at your own clumsy mending. The places of anger are frightening for many people in our society. Unlike the places of denial, we usually know we are angry and this makes us very uncomfortable, for many of us were taught, as children, that being angry is bad. Maybe we hit a brother or sister with a toy truck and, when asked why we had done such a thing, we explained that we were mad at the person. Unfortunately few of us were then told that it was all right to be mad at someone, but not all right to hit him or her with a truck. Instead we were told that we were a bad child for even being angry. And so we learned, many of us very early in life, not to let anyone know that we were angry.

Many of us were also taught that as bad as it was to be angry when there was a reason, it was really unacceptable to be angry with someone for something that was not the person's fault. People have told me again and again how ashamed they are because they are angry at the child who died. "It wasn't his or her fault," they tell me, "so I have no right to be angry." I think this is one of the reasons some bereaved persons get so angry with physicians or nurses, or other medical personnel. I am not talking about those instances when some person really is at fault, but those instances when that individual just happened to be there at the time. Getting angry at such persons is usually considered inappropriate, but more excusable than getting angry at an innocent person who has died.

Anger is a feeling, and all feelings and thoughts are all right. It is what we do with our feelings and thoughts that matters. Keep reminding yourself that it is all right to feel angry. Perhaps you are angry at your loved one for dying. Others tell you that this does not make sense. Your loved one is not to blame. Being angry does not have to make sense. Anger is a feeling, not some sort of logical exercise.

Many people in my part of the country, especially older people, have trouble with being angry at God. One elderly woman once confided in me that she hoped God would never know how really angry she was at Him for letting her husband die and leaving her so alone. This dear woman was so afraid God would realize how angry she was that she quit going to church. I asked her if she really wanted to place her destiny in the hands of a Being that knew so little. She thought about it and then said, "You're right. God knows." Relieved of trying to keep this terrible secret from God, she cried out both her anguish and her rage to God. I really do not think God was any the worse for this, and the woman certainly felt much better. She returned to her church and the comfort that it could provide her.

Anger directed at God may be one of the most authentic forms of prayer. I remember sitting one afternoon with a man who was angry at God for allowing his son to be killed. Given a safe place and permission to vent his feelings, he poured out his rage to God. He was a powerful man and it seemed to me as though his screams rose through the ceiling and into the heavens above. I thought about the many times I had gone to church and looked at my watch repeatedly, going over in my mind all I wanted to do as soon as I could return home. I attended church, said my prayers, behaved in an appropriate way, but my thoughts were on other matters. This man's whole being, his total attention, was focused on God. The more fully prayer is entered into, the more powerful the prayer. This man was in total communion with God; his screams to God were a magnificent testimony to that communion.

Just as there are many places of denial, there are many places of anger. You may get angry when you see the tear, angry when you realize how big it is, angry when you think about all that will have to be done to mend it, angry when you cannot find the right needle or thread, angry when your stitches do not hold, angry at having to mend in the first place, even angry at being so angry. Perhaps you are getting angry at what is written in this book or angry at me for writing it. It is all right to be angry. There does not have to be a reason; just being angry because you are angry is reason enough. What you do with your anger is what matters. If you must have a reason, just remember your fabric is torn. That is reason enough. In another chapter are some suggestions for ways to work through your anger. For now, there are still some other places to consider.

DEPRESSION

Because we were often told when we were children that getting angry is bad, or wrong, or even sinful, many of us learned to hide angry feelings from others. You may have become so skilled at doing this that you even hide your angry feelings from yourself. This can lead to depression. Just as with denial and anger, however, there are different places called depression. One is a place you may enter if you hide your angry feelings from yourself. Before talking about this place, however, there is another place of depression—clinical depression. This type of depression must always be considered first, because it can have serious consequences if this is where you are. Loss can affect a person physically as well as emotionally. I always recommend that anyone who has lost an important person in his or her life see a physician as soon as possible for a physical checkup.

Loss affects the body's chemical balance and medication may be called for. Relatives and friends, no matter how well intentioned, are not qualified to recognize these changes and prescribe the appropriate medicine. Medicines that might have been helpful in earlier times, even over-the-counter medicines, may cause serious problems during times of stress. Grief is stressful. If you are going to take any medicine, you need expert advice.

Look for a physician who will allow you to talk about your loss or who is at least aware of your loss and accepts it as important.[1] Some physicians cannot cope with loss, their own or anyone else's. You need one who will recognize that your loss is an important factor in your life and that your grief is warranted. That way you will receive medication intended to help you in your mending process, not medication to mask your pain so that you will not upset others, including your physician, with your anguish.

The need for medication is not a sign of weakness. You cannot mend your fabric when you spend night after night with no sleep or when you are unable to eat. Just make certain that the medication is intended to help you move through the mending process. You do not want to take medicine that is intended to cause you to put your mending down and pretend that your fabric is either not really torn or that the tear is so small and insignificant that little or no mending is needed.

The place of depression that you enter because of suppressed anger is different from clinical depression. Medication will not help you here. The only way to move out of this place is to affirm and release the anger itself. For some people, this is one of the most difficult aspects of mending, and thus, may require very special needles and threads. You may need assistance in both finding, as well as using, these needles and threads. Sometimes persons who have been through the mending process themselves can provide direction. It is possible that you may need to work with a professional seamstress or tailor. This is what seeking professional help really is all about. How to go about finding these people is discussed in a later chapter. There is yet another place you may have been in, or may be in now, that is often confused with depression. This is the place of sadness.

---

[1] It is possible that your local hospital chaplain or someone in social services at the hospital can assist you in finding such a physician.

SADNESS

Just as with anger, many of us were forbidden as children to enter the place of sadness as well. When you were a child, were you ever told to stop crying? When I was a little girl, I was told that crying made me ugly. If you are male, you were probably told that crying was sissy. The adults in your childhood also may have told you that you really had nothing to cry about. Your loss was not that big a loss, or it really did not hurt you that much. How did they know? It was your loss, not their loss; it was your pain, not their pain. I remember being told when I was a child that if I did not quit crying that very instant, I would be given something to cry about. Thus, whenever I entered a place of sadness, I was pushed or goaded out of it by some adult. I tried my best to stay away from this place. If you were ever told not to cry, you may have learned to avoid this place also.

It is all right to be sad when your fabric has been torn. It is also all right to cry. Indeed, it may be very important that you spend time crying as well as just sitting in a place of sadness. I often tell the men who come to me that maybe it is true that boys do not cry, but real men certainly do! I facilitate a support group for men living with AIDS and many of these men have told me that they are ashamed to admit that they have been "sitting on the pity pot." I always tell them, "Hey, it's your pity pot. Sit on it as long as you want." Part of mending is just sitting and looking at your fabric and remembering what it looked like before it was torn and wondering if you will ever be able to do anything with it again. Just sitting with your fabric and crying may be the very best thing you can do when you are not certain how you feel or what you want to do at the time. You may also need to cry in order to be better prepared physically to mend your fabric.

Counselors who work with grieving persons have long recognized that crying helps release tension. Now researchers tell us that crying does more than relieve physical tension. Crying removes chemicals from the body that have built up as a result of emotional stress [2]. These chemicals are toxic and will cause physical harm if they are not eliminated from the body. Crying does this for us naturally. So the place of sadness is more than just a place you may enter at one time or another during the mending process; it is a place you may need to seek out from time to time. Since this place may have been off limits to you when you were a child, you may need assistance in finding it as well as help in remaining in it until it is time (your time) to move to a different place. Just keep in mind that sadness, like anger, is a feeling and all feelings are all right. It is what you do with your feelings that is important.

RELIEF

Although the place of relief was probably never forbidden when you were a child, feeling relieved causes problems for many bereaved persons. Relief, however, is a place people often enter when death follows a long illness. The paths that lead to this place vary. You may be relieved that the pain and suffering of your loved one is over; you may be physically and emotionally exhausted and relieved that at long last you can sleep without jumping up at the least little sound. You may be relieved that the very thing you have dreaded for so long, the actual death itself, is over.

You may even be relieved that the person who died is dead for other reasons. Perhaps this person made you uncomfortable, or frightened you, or kept your life in turmoil. This is especially true in suicide. In her wonderful little book, *That Nothing Be Wasted,* written after the death of her son by suicide, Mary Langford writes:

> Not all deaths are unexpected, or unwelcome. Even suicides bring relief to some, especially when the relationship had grown destructive. When the cause of their emotional upheaval is removed, many family members breathe sighs of relief after the suicide, often bypassing the emotional flood that usually follows shock [3, p. 49].

I remember reading this passage after a member of my family killed himself. I used to dread this person's threatening phone calls and I was so relieved that I never had to pick up the phone and hear his threats again. I felt so guilty about feeling relief, however, and it was such a comfort to know others felt as I did and that it was all right to feel that way.

There is also a feeling of relief that at long last one can get on with one's mending. Caretakers often tell me that they dread the grief they know they will have to deal with when the person they love finally dies. It is as though their fabric is in the process of being torn and they must wait until the tear is completed in order to begin mending. Whatever the reason, relief is a feeling, just like anger and sadness, and just as it is all right to feel angry or sad, it is all right to feel relief.

FEAR

Another place in which I often find bereaved persons is the place of fear. As I go over these places in my workshops, I am constantly reminded that many of us were forbidden to enter most of them when we were children. This is true of anger and sadness. It is true of fear as well. Were you ever told not to be afraid? Being called a coward was one of the worst things you could be called when I was growing up. I was often told, "There really is nothing to be afraid of. Your fear is all in your mind." But the imagined tiger that lurked under my bed when I was a child was very real to me, and I was afraid. I tried to be brave and not let anyone know I was afraid, but I often lay in my bed at night listening to the growls of the tiger that lay in wait, ready to devour me if I slept.

And on the playground at school, other children called me a "scaredy cat" when I would not climb to the top of the monkey bars. I often wondered which was worse, being called a "scaredy cat" or the horrible dizziness I felt the few times I did climb up the bars. People often share with me how ashamed they are of feeling so afraid both during and following their loved one's illness. Fear, however, is a place many enter at such times. You may fear what you think may happen to you now that your loved one has died. You may fear the unknown. Feeling afraid is difficult enough. You do not need to fear feeling afraid as well.

JEALOUSY

Denial, anger, depression, sadness, relief, and fear are only some of the places bereaved persons enter in the grieving process. These are, however, places I most frequently find bereaved persons. There are also other places some people enter at one time or another. Jealousy is one of these. You may be jealous of the person who died. This is reasonable. His or her problems are over; your problems seem to be just beginning. Bereaved persons also tell me they are jealous of others who are busily getting on with their lives. Sometimes these persons try to encourage or even push the bereaved person to join them in activities.

One mother told me that she would get angry with her sister for trying to get her to go shopping. At the same time, she said, she was so jealous of her sister for being able to even think about shopping. As much as she wanted to avoid the place of anger, she felt that the place of jealousy was even worse. Being in the place of jealousy, however, can be very helpful when you are mending. When you are envious of another person, you are focusing for the moment on how your life might be rather than how it is. Jealousy, then, can inspire you to get on with your mending. It can help you exit a place of sadness, not because you should exit this place, but because you want to leave it, at least for a time, in order to do something you would like to do.

ACCEPTANCE

The last place I want to mention is really not a place at all, although it is often mistaken for one. This is acceptance. I often invite people who have experienced a great loss to come to the university where I teach and speak to my Death and Dying class. One year a woman whose husband had died several years previously came to speak to my students about being elderly and widowed. She talked about what it was like to lose the person who had been her great love, her best friend, her life's companion. He was ill for a long time before he died and she spoke about her struggle to become involved once more with life, to meet new friends, and undertake new activities. One student was so taken with this woman's story and how far she had come since her husband's death that he said to her in awe, "You've reached acceptance!" She smiled and responded, "Oh my dear child, acceptance is not a point of arrival; it's a process." And so it is.

Many times bereaved persons move out of a particular place or allow others to push them out because they think, like my student, that acceptance is also a place and the sooner they reach this place, the better it will be for everyone. Acceptance is not a place; it is a process. As we mend our fabrics, we will weave in and out of acceptance, in and out, in and out. The woman who spoke to my class shared how she first had to accept how very lonely she was before she could begin to reach out and open up to others. She then had to accept that she would have to explore different ways of reaching out to others. Perhaps you have been trying to mend your fabric with old needles and threads and you finally accept that you will need to search for new ones. You may try someone else's needle, and finally accept that the best one for you has been right there in your own sewing basket the whole time. Just accepting the place you are in at any given moment is part of the process. It is all right to be angry or sad or relieved. You may not like feeling a certain feeling; it is all right to feel that way. Ultimately you may accept that your mending is done, at least for a time, and allow yourself to try embroidering again.

Through the years I have asked my students to try to define acceptance after listening to what bereaved persons have shared with them in class. One wrote, "Arriving at acceptance is not like arriving in New York. It is more like arriving in New York; then New York moves." Another suggested:

> Acceptance is like going to the beach and getting your feet wet in the surf. It's cold so you back off. You go out again, getting wet to the waist, and then back off again. Finally you go in all the way. It's a process. [Eventually] whatever you are facing and going through no longer holds power over you.

You may never accept your loss in that you no longer feel pain when you think about your loved one who died. Some deaths are never accepted in this sense. Newly bereaved parents often ask those in the support group who have been mending for some time, "Will the pain ever go away?" The reply is always the same. "No, but it will become a part of you, not something that controls you." Some tears can never be mended completely. They can be mended, however, so that the tear is no longer all that you see when you look at your fabric.

Perhaps you are in a place I have not mentioned. If you feel that this is the right place for you to be in, stay there. If you are not certain, the following questions may help you. Can you learn anything about your fabric in the place you are in? What can you learn about your tear? Are there needles and threads that you need to look for? Can you find them in that place or do you need to move to another place? How did you come to be in that place? Have you ever been there before? If so, how did you leave the last time you were there? Did you leave because you were ready to leave or were you pushed or pulled out by someone? Is there some other place you would like to go? Take your time. Your fabric is torn. You may enter many places, some many times, before your mending is done.

There are, however, two places that you want to avoid while mending your torn fabric. Although these two places are easy to stumble into if your fabric is torn, you cannot rest or mend in either of them. They are also places where you can get stuck if you do not recognize where you are and how you came to be there. Before we talk about these places, however, repeat the following lines several times.

All of my feelings are ok.

All of my thoughts are ok.

It is what I do with my feelings and thoughts that matters.

REFERENCES

1. E. Kübler-Ross, *On Death and Dying* (Preface), Macmillan, New York, 1967.
2. G. Levoy, Tears That Speak, *Psychology Today, 22*:7/8, pp. 8, 10, 1988.
3. M. Langford, *That Nothing Be Wasted,* New Hope, Birmingham, Alabama, 1988.

Chapter 3

PLACES TO AVOID

Denial, anger, sadness, relief, fear, and jealousy are all places you may have been in at one time or another. Perhaps you are in one of these places as you read this book. These are neither good places nor bad places. They are simply places, and you may need to remain in one of them for some time or return to one or more at some later time in order to learn more about your fabric, your tear or tears, and the mending you need to do. Some are places in which you will be able to work on your tear; others are places in which you can rest before beginning or resuming your mending.

There will probably be other places in your journey that I have not mentioned. Grief does not come with a road map or a timetable. No two people have the same fabric; no two people have the same tears; and no two people will mend tears in exactly the same way. You will have to decide whether it is best to remain in a place for a time before moving on or whether to return to a place you have visited before.

There are, however, two places to avoid. If you do find yourself in one of these places, exit as quickly as possible. One of these is the place of guilt; the other is the place of shame. Guilt and shame are very different from the feelings we talked about in the last chapter. Denial, anger, sadness, relief, fear, and jealousy are natural feelings. We may learn how to express these feelings or even if we can express them. We can learn when or if these feelings are appropriate. Guilt and shame are not natural feelings. We learn to feel guilt and shame. Before we can feel either guilt or shame, we have to first learn to think about ourself in some way. Thus, in order to enter a place of guilt, we have to first believe that we have done something wrong. In order to enter the place of shame, we have to first believe that we are a bad person.

People are especially vulnerable following the loss of someone who was very important in their life. The struggle to keep the fragments of a badly torn fabric from further disintegration is in itself overwhelming. A woman whose daughter died following an automobile accident once shared with me that she felt as if her whole being might suddenly shatter into tiny little pieces and evaporate into the universe. As a result of this fragmentation, bereaved persons often move from place to place, sometimes very rapidly. This rapid movement from place to place is both confusing and frightening. For days, weeks, and even months following a great loss in your life, you may find it difficult to even know what you are feeling at any given moment. You certainly do not know what you will be feeling a few minutes later.

Bereaved persons often ask me if I think they are going crazy. In a real sense a bereaved person is crazy. Sanity is dependent upon living in an ordered world. When you have lost someone very important to you, there is no order in your world. There is only chaos. You may not be able to stop crying. You may have trouble falling asleep, or you may want to sleep most of the time. Food has no taste.

I particularly remember a young woman whose five-year-old son had recently died from a surgery the parents believed would be routine. She asked me if I thought she would ever stop crying. It hurt her to breathe; she felt that at any moment she might explode into a million pieces. It is difficult for a person in this state of chaos to even see his or her fabric. There is only this enormous hole that seems to grow larger and larger with each passing moment. In times of such chaos, it is very easy to fall into or be pushed into a place of guilt or shame.

There are at least four different paths that lead to both of these places. Sometimes these paths overlap, but the origin of each path differs. Knowing where these paths begin may help you understand how you might have come to a place of guilt or a place of shame and how you can avoid these places in the future. The beginning of one of the paths to guilt or shame may be in your cultural background. A second path may be traced to your personal history, particularly your childhood. A third path to guilt or shame may spring from how other people define your loss. Finally, a fourth path may stem from aspects of the relationship you had with the person who died. Sometimes it is difficult to recognize which of these paths led you to a place of guilt or shame. Thus, it is important to look at all four possibilities: your cultural background, your own personal history, how other people define your loss, and your relationship with the person who died. Perhaps this will help you avoid a place of either guilt or shame or help you to climb out if you are already there.

CULTURAL BACKGROUND

Our culture is where we get our ideas about what our world looks like, the part we play in this world, what we ought to do or not do, and what we have a right to expect from others. Most of the time we are unaware of our culture, especially if we are surrounded by persons who share the same cultural background. We rarely think that we are behaving in a particular way because we have learned to behave that way. When someone does not behave in an expected way, however, we turn to those who share our own cultural background for affirmation that the person did not behave as he or she should have. Mourning is that part of our cultural background that has to do with loss, grief, and grief work.

Mourning is a set of instructions you receive from your culture that tells you how to think and feel about the tears in your fabric, and how to mend them. When you use the word "normal," you are probably describing how your culture defines something for you. Thus, you may think that it is normal for all people to cry at funerals, or you may think that it is normal for only certain persons to cry at funerals but not for others. You may think that crying is acceptable behavior, but sobbing or wailing is not. Whether or not one is supposed to cry at funerals and how much crying is acceptable are examples of mourning rules or customs. Mourning rules and customs, however, differ considerably across cultures. In some cultures crying is expected; in others, crying is permitted; in still others, crying is considered to be a sign of weakness or disrespect for the deceased.

Whether or not to cry is only one of many mourning rules. In one culture it may be proper for the person who has died to be buried as quickly as possible. In another culture waiting several days or even a week or more is appropriate. The Toraja people of Sulawesi, an island in the Indonesian archipelago, may wait a year or more to bury a person [1]. These people think it is terrible to bury someone before all the necessary things have been done or acquired to perform the funeral rites correctly. The body of the deceased person remains at home until all is in readiness. We would probably define a person or family who did this in our society as mentally ill. The Toraja people define it as the proper way of doing things and the appropriate way to show respect for someone who has died.

How and by whom the body is prepared and how and where the body is buried also differ widely across cultures. Whether or not there is a wake or a visitation before burial services, who is expected to come, and what that person is expected to do or not do are also mourning rules or customs and differ from culture to culture.

I grew up in a small town in Georgia. Friends and business associates were expected to go to the home of the person who died. The immediate family usually remained secluded in a back room. Only very close friends or business acquaintances were taken to this room. There were always several older women who somehow knew which persons should be taken to speak to the family. These women invited you into the family's room. If you were not invited to visit with the family, you simply viewed the body of the person who had died and signed the register. It would have been considered very inappropriate to ask to see the family.

Shortly after I moved to southern Louisiana, a colleague's mother died and my husband and I went to the funeral home to pay our respects. I was greatly embarrassed when I suddenly found myself in the middle of the immediate family, meeting all but my colleague for the first time. I felt as though I had done something terrible and wondered for some time how I had happened to blunder into the wrong room or enter it at the wrong time. Only later did I learn that in southern Louisiana the immediate family remains in the room with the body and speaks to every person who comes to honor the deceased person. At first I thought such behavior was odd. I have lived in Louisiana for over twenty years and I am now comfortable with this way of doing things. I have even begun to think the way we did it in Georgia was not as "normal" as the way it is done in southern Louisiana. Neither way, however, is right or wrong. What is important is that there are different ways of doing things and we are most comfortable when things are done the way we are accustomed to having them done.

In your great grandparents' time, or perhaps even in your grandparents' time, there was usually no problem with how things were done. People who lived in the same community generally agreed on how to do many things, particularly with respect to important life events. Since death is an important life event, there were definite ways of doing things associated with this event. Within each community, that community's way was considered normal. It is very comforting to know that we are thinking or feeling or behaving in a "normal" manner.

In the times in which we live, however, the best or even an acceptable way of doing things is rarely clear. Most of us live in communities made up of people from different parts of the United States, even different parts of the world. I may want things done the way they did them in Georgia. You may want them done the way they were done somewhere else. We are following different cultural guidelines. As a result, neither of us is certain just how we should be doing things.

Perhaps you think you should have waited longer for the funeral or had it sooner. Perhaps you think you should have done something else or done it differently. And suddenly you are in a place of guilt or shame. You are not there because you did something wrong; you are there because you think you did something you should not have done or you think you did not do something you should have done. This, of course, happens in other areas of our lives as well. Usually we think about it for a time and then decide that next time we might do it differently and let it go at that. When you have lost someone very dear to you, however, there is not going to be a next time. There was only this one time and you have lost forever the opportunity to do it properly. You may feel so guilty; you may feel so ashamed.

If you are in one of these places, it is important to remember that there is no *one* right or wrong way to do things. There is only a particular culture's way of doing things and you are probably trying to follow the rules and customs of several, perhaps even numerous, cultures. People in traditional communities had only one way of doing things. Having a set way of doing things does not take away the pain of loss, but it does provide an orderly way of moving through a very difficult time in your life. If you planned the funeral for your loved one, you were faced with many decisions and you had to make a number of choices. Because most of us live today in multicultural communities, you probably lived through a time of enormous stress without a clear set of rules to follow.

Allow yourself to feel angry, at yourself or others, for not doing things differently. Allow yourself to feel sad for lost opportunities. These feelings, if acknowledged, will run their course. Feeling guilty or ashamed will not get you anywhere. These places are like deep pits of mud. The longer you sit in one of them, the deeper you will sink and the harder it will be to pull yourself out. The best thing to do is climb out right now, even if it means jumping into a place of anger or a place of sadness. When you have done the grief work you need to do, you will emerge from these places with at least some of your mending done. You cannot get any mending done sitting in a place of guilt or shame, and you certainly will not get any rest.

PERSONAL HISTORY

Another path that leads toward both guilt and shame originates in individual or personal experience. This path, of course, often overlaps with your cultural background. Sometimes, you learned to do things or think about things a certain way because that is how people in your particular community did things or thought about things. Sometimes you learned to do things or think about things a certain way because of the particular people you encountered during your childhood, especially your family.

For example, perhaps you were taught that crying was for babies. Maybe your friends were taught this also. Maybe this notion was limited to your family. Regardless, you were taught that crying was something to be ashamed of. Now you have lost someone very dear to you and it is difficult, perhaps even impossible, for you not to cry. Whenever you begin to cry, however, you recall old messages you received as a child and you feel ashamed of yourself for "acting like a baby." Someone may be telling you now that your sad face makes others unhappy. "You should try to get yourself together and not dwell on your loss," they tell you. Now you not only feel ashamed for crying, you feel guilty about making others unhappy. You are following a path right out of your childhood into a place of guilt and/or shame.

Perhaps you were told as a child that getting angry was a sign of weakness. As a result, you filed away in your memory the message, "Strong people do not get angry." Now you sit with your torn fabric and the rage within you threatens to erupt and you are not strong enough to contain it. You are ashamed of such weakness. You cannot even look at your fabric, because to do so evokes even more anger and, thus, more shame. You are not a weak person. You have a badly torn fabric. You think you are weak, however, because you learned to think this way when you were very young and it is very difficult to unlearn early thinking. It is particularly difficult to unlearn early thinking when your life is so out of control, when you are in so much pain. You may be thinking, "Perhaps these other people are right. Maybe I am just a weak person. If I were a strong person, I would be better able to control my anger or not cry so much."

Notice what is happening to you! The muddy mire of guilt or shame is pulling you down deeper and deeper. Recognize where you are and try to climb out. If you are in very deep, you may need professional help to get out. We will talk about how to find this help later in another chapter. For now, just remember that feeling angry or sad are natural responses to loss. It is what you do with these feelings that matters. And what you were taught as a child or what others say you ought to feel or do may not be best for you at this time in your life. Your fabric is different from anyone else's fabric and the tear in your fabric is the only one of its kind.

Others may suggest how you should mend your fabric. You may find their suggestions helpful. There may be needles and threads from your childhood that will be useful. There is, however, no right or wrong way to mend. Ultimately, you will have to decide which needles and threads are best for you. You will never be able to find the right needles and threads or to decide how to use them if you are sitting in the slippery muck of guilt or shame.

How we ought to feel and what we are supposed to do with our feelings are only two things we are taught, either through our culture in general or through those individuals who cared for us, or at least were responsible for our care, when we were children. We also learned how to think about loss. Remember when you were little and you did not get to do something you wanted to do. Did anyone ever tell you that it was not that important, so stop crying? But it was important to you. Whatever it was that you wanted to do, you really wanted to do it. And when you could not do it, you were disappointed. Perhaps you lost something of value to you or someone took something that you valued away from you and once again, you were told that losing that thing was not that big a loss and to stop crying. But it was a big loss for you. Maybe it did not seem important or valuable to anyone else, but it was to you.

One of my students told me that when she was a little girl she had a doll she loved very much. She always slept with this doll at night. She shared her secrets with her doll and when she was afraid or sad, she would hold her doll very tightly and this always made her feel better. One day, her mother decided to clean house and get rid of things that were no longer useful. The doll was old and tattered. Most of her hair was gone and one eye no longer closed and so the mother threw the doll in the garbage. When my student came home from school, she discovered that her doll was missing and looked for her everywhere she could think to look. Finally she asked her mother to help her look for her doll. It was then that she learned that her doll was gone forever.

She was devastated at the loss at the time, and the memory of that loss still caused her pain. As she sat in my office, she wept for her doll. She shared that her mother kept telling her that the doll was old and losing it was not such a big loss. She was told to grow up and act like a big girl. She was too old to play with dolls anyway. She told me she had feared for a long time that something was wrong with her because she could not forget losing her doll. She was ashamed of "carrying on so." That afternoon, she climbed out of the place of shame and moved first into the place of sadness and then the place of anger, then back into sadness. At long last, she had begun her mending. All I had done for her was to affirm that losing her doll was a loss worth grieving. I had given her permission to grieve.

This young woman was in pain, but she could not move through the pain toward healing because allowing herself to hurt because of the loss of her doll created another pain, the pain of shame. We are social beings which means we look to others for affirmation that who we are and what we are doing is acceptable. If the loss which prompted the pain is not recognized, or as in the case of my student, the loss is trivialized, our pain is considered inappropriate by others. When there is no affirmation of loss and, thus, pain, the person who hurts begins to think that something is wrong with him or her.

Allowing the loss to justify the pain is really going about it backwards. It is true that the tear in your fabric precipitated your pain. How the tear is defined by others, however, cannot be the deciding issue in determining if your pain is appropriate. We need to begin with the pain, not the tear. If there is pain, there is a tear. If the pain is great, the tear is a large tear. You know if you are hurting. If you are, there is a tear in your fabric, and this tear will have to be mended or it will continue to control, or at least interfere with, your life. If your pain is intense, your tear is large.

We are social beings, however, and affirmation from others is important. This is particularly true in difficult or chaotic times. When we do not receive affirmation of our loss and pain, it is very easy to fall into a place of guilt or shame. For many of us it is difficult enough to admit to ourselves that we are angry or sad or afraid. It is even more difficult to have these feelings for no reason, or at least no reason that is accepted or recognized by others. Grief that others do not acknowledge is called *disenfranchised grief*. A third path to guilt and/or shame, then, begins when others do not acknowledge our tear.

HOW OTHER PEOPLE DEFINE YOUR LOSS

Family and friends often do not acknowledge the terrible loss to the parent when there is a miscarriage, or stillbirth, or when a baby dies shortly after birth. The parents may be told to forget about what has happened. They can have other children. Although other children may add wonderful colors and patterns to a parent's fabric, other children cannot undo the tear or tears left by the child who died. A parent who has suffered a miscarriage needs time to mend his or her torn fabric, but it is difficult to work on your mending when others are telling you that you do not have a real tear, or that it is only a small nick.

In a very early miscarriage, the father may not have bonded with the baby.[1] When this happens, the mother may be the only one whose fabric is greatly torn. Her husband and other family members, as well as friends, may console her for a short time, but they are convinced that she will feel better if she just forgets about what happened. The mother may have to put her mending aside or mend alone. If she mends alone, she may be pushed into a place of guilt or shame. If she tries to ignore her tear, however, it will go unmended and perhaps tear even more.

Advances in medical technology in the area of infertility have created a new kind of disenfranchised grief. For those parents unable to have children, a number of possibilities now offer hope. One of these is the in-vitro fertilization process in which eggs or ovum are harvested from the mother, placed in a petri dish, and fertilized by the father's or a donor's sperm. A few days later, the fertilized eggs are placed in the mother's uterus. In the meantime, the mother is given drugs that cause her body to mimic pregnancy in order to facilitate the implantation of the fertilized eggs. If this implantation takes place, a baby or babies result. In many cases the fertilized eggs do not implant. Because of the drugs, however, the mother feels pregnant. This is only a chemical pregnancy. If there is no implantation, no actual

---

[1] It is certainly possible that although the father did not bond with the baby in the way that the mother did, he bonded with the "idea" of a child. If so, his fabric is also torn.

pregnancy took place. At least this is what the couple are told by others. As a result, they are not even granted the few days of consolation accorded parents who lose their babies through miscarriage. There was no pregnancy, thus no tear, thus no need for grief. These parents must either deny their grief or grieve alone.

Of course these parents have spent months preparing for this procedure. Each step has been one more phase on an emotional roller coaster. They may have waited months or even years before they were even accepted into a program. The eggs were successfully harvested. Fertilization took place, and the fertilized eggs were placed in the mother's uterus. The couple's long-awaited dream of having a baby seemed so close to coming true. All the physical signs of pregnancy were there. And then they are told it was only a chemical pregnancy. Two fabrics are ripped; his and hers. This is terrible enough to bear, but then they are told that neither of their fabrics is really torn. She was not even pregnant. There was no baby.

Actually there were two babies, the baby that existed in her heart and the baby that existed in his. Parents who have been through this process have shared with me how angry they were that no one would recognize their loss. Often they add that they feel guilt or shame for being so angry. Because a loss is disenfranchised does not mean that there is no tear in your fabric. It means that you will have to mend alone or look for someone who will sit with you while you mend. It will take a great deal of determination and courage on your part to mend your fabric when no one will even acknowledge that your fabric is torn. Your pain, however, is proof that your fabric is torn. If your fabric is torn, you have a right, indeed a need, to mend it.

Bereaved persons are often told they should be grateful; it could be worse or there are others in worse shape. One young woman told me that following a hysterectomy, she grieved for the children she would never have. She was told that she should be grateful for the one child she did have. She felt so guilty for not feeling grateful. She loved her child, but she also grieved for the additional children she wanted but could no longer have.

Every time someone told her she should feel grateful for the child she had, she felt both guilt and shame. Sometimes we stumble into guilt or shame. Sometimes we allow others to push us into one of these places.

Even when there is affirmation from others that your fabric is torn, there may be inconsistent messages about acceptable ways to mend it and how long the mending should take. One woman told me that people were very kind to her following her little boy's death from a bicycle accident. Family and friends brought food, took care of her other children, sat with her while she wept. After a few months, however, they wanted her to "get over it." She was chided on more than one occasion for ruining family get-togethers with "her long face." She tried to hide her pain when she was around others, but her thoughts were always on her little boy.

One afternoon, however, she and her husband attended a wedding ceremony and the reception that followed. She had not wanted to go, but family members had pressured her. She "owed" it to the bride and groom and their parents to attend. There was a dance, and for a brief moment, she forgot her loss. Perhaps she was in a place of denial. She certainly needed and deserved a time of rest. Regardless, her husband asked her to dance and she accepted. She had only taken a few steps when she noticed the shocked glances of some of her relatives. The very same people who had accused her of ruining family gatherings now criticized her for dancing. She told me that she felt that she had somehow betrayed her child. She wept as she said, "No matter what I do, I'm always wrong."

This is a good illustration of being "damned if you do and damned if you don't." Your loss may not be defined as worthy of grief. Even if your loss is defined as a great loss, ideas about how you should respond to such a loss may vary. It is as though you are in a car you do not know how to drive. You are lost; you have no road map, and the road signs direct you first in one direction and then in another. If you add to this scenario that you are in terrible pain, you have a picture of what grieving a terrible loss is like in a multicultural society. It is very easy to fall or be pushed into a place of guilt or shame.

YOUR RELATIONSHIP WITH THE
PERSON WHO DIED

There is also a fourth path that may lead toward guilt and/or shame. This path originates in the relationship you had with the person who died. Relationships that are important to us are rarely either all positive or all negative. We usually get the angriest with those we love the most. We disappoint them; they disappoint us. When death is sudden and unexpected, we are left with all the "if onlys." If only I had told him I loved him, if only I had told her I was sorry for something I did or did not do. If only, if only, if only. If the person was ill for a long time there may be other regrets. If only I had been more patient; if only I had done more. If only, if only, if only.

People often ask me which death is worse, sudden death or death following a long illness. If the person was important to you, either kind of death is devastating. Neither kind of death is worse or less painful than the other one. Sudden death and death following a long illness are, however, quite different and the remorse following the death tends to be different. If the person died suddenly, there are probably things you said or did not say that you wish now you had said or left unsaid. The physical shock of losing someone suddenly can be catastrophic. We will talk about the impact of sudden death in more detail in a later chapter. Regardless of the type of death, remorse can lead to guilt or shame.

If you knew death was near, you may have said what you wanted to say. You may still wonder, though, if you did all to comfort him or her that you could have done. If only you could prepare one more special dish to tempt a diminished appetite, fluff a pillow, place a cool cloth on a fevered brow, or hold a hand. These regrets are part of the tear in your fabric. They are the frayed edges. The more regrets, the more ragged the tear. These edges may need to be repaired before you can attend to the tear itself. You will not be able to mend them if you are sitting in the muck of guilt and shame.

There is nothing more that you can do in a physical way for this person you loved. And you hurt. You may feel relieved that this person you loved is not suffering any more. You may be angry at your loved one for dying and leaving you. You may be sad because you miss this person so much. You may feel lonely or frightened when you think of the days to come, of long evenings alone, of holidays without him or her. You may feel many different feelings and sometimes you may feel different feelings at the same time. You have a right to your feelings, for you have lost someone very special to you. Honor your feelings, even if no one else does. Honor your pain, even if no one else will acknowledge that your fabric is torn.

You cannot honor your feelings, you cannot truly grieve your loved one, if you allow "shoulda, coulda, woulda" thoughts to get between you and your feelings and between you and the person who died. These thoughts, however, are often difficult to push away, because they are often true. You are a human being; you were not and are not perfect. You did not do all that you should have done (shoulda), or could have done (coulda), or would have done (woulda) if you had only known then what you know now. If only, if only. It is so easy to fall into a place of guilt or shame. Perhaps you felt anger toward the person before he or she died, but pushed these feelings aside during the illness that preceded death. Now these angry feelings emerge and frighten you. You are ashamed about the way you felt then and now. You may be angry about being alone. Others may tell you to think about the person who died. Surely you would not want him or her to suffer any more. Well, what about you? You are tired of suffering too. And then you feel shame for thinking such thoughts.

Fortunately, there are signs that warn us that we are either about to stumble or to be pushed into one of these places or that we are already in one of them. Whether it is our cultural background, our personal history, other people's cultural background or personal histories, or the relationship between us and the person we have lost, there are signs that warn us that we are in or near the places of guilt or shame.

Earlier we defined mourning as what others tell us or what we have learned to tell ourselves about our tears, how to think and feel about our tears, and how to mend them. As children, we were told by others that we should or ought to feel or think or behave a certain way or that we should not or ought not to feel or think or behave a particular way. Listen carefully to what other people are saying to you and to what you are saying to yourself. The words, "should" and "ought," are signs that you may be close to or already in a place of guilt or shame.

There is also another word to listen out for as well, the little word, "but." You will find this little word in sentences like "It's all right for you to cry, but not for so long," or "It's all right for you to go to the cemetery, but not every day." Listening out for the "shoulds," "oughts," and "buts" can help you avoid falling or being pushed into guilt and shame.

Avoiding the places of guilt and/or shame are especially difficult if there is any question of fault. Western cultures tend to be cause oriented. We want to know why something happened and we are rarely content until we find out the answer or at least an answer that satisfies us. This is, after all, the force that drives scientific inquiry. We want to know why; we are taught to ask why. When something bad happens to someone, we want to know why for another reason as well. If we know why, perhaps we can avoid having something bad happen to us.

I am always amazed when attending wakes to hear some of the questions people ask. "How did he or she die?" This question is closely followed by others. "What did he do?" "What did she not do?" And finally, "Didn't anyone recognize what was happening?" These questions are probably asked with little or no thought about their impact on the bereaved. Often, however, they are questions a bereaved person is also asking. Was there something I should have done or should not have done? Was there something I should have noticed? Blame pushes us immediately into guilt or shame. I once heard a priest say, "If you are truly to blame, fall on your knees and ask forgiveness of your God and of your fellow humans. If not, let it go." Again, allow yourself to be angry at yourself for something you did or did not do. Allow yourself to be sad. Try to stay away from the places of guilt and shame. Climb out if you are already there. Seek professional help if you find this too difficult to do alone.

Some of the messages that we have learned or hear that push us toward these places may be very subtle and difficult to recognize. One night at a Compassionate Friends meeting, a young bereaved mother suddenly screamed, "Quit saying I lost my child; my child died!" The room became very still as she shared that every time she heard the word, "lost," it was as though she were being accused of leaving her child in the grocery store somewhere between the vegetables and the meat counter. Following her outburst, several bereaved parents agreed that the word, "lost," bothered them as well. It implied they were somehow at fault. One parent said that parents are supposed to take care of their children. A good parent does not "lose" his or her child. Most parents feel guilty to some degree if their child dies. There is so much pain; guilt is usually an undeserved burden.

Blame as defined by your culture may push you toward guilt or shame. Messages you received when you were a child may push you as well. Perhaps as a child you were often blamed for one thing or another. Perhaps you were given more responsibility than you were capable of handling at that time. There may have been additional pressures on you as well. Perhaps there was a time when you were at fault and your family has never forgotten. Whatever the reason, you have learned to blame yourself if things do not go as you think they should. If so, you do not need anyone to push you into a place of guilt or shame. You jump into one of these places when anything goes wrong in your life or the lives of people you care about. Whatever the reason, it is time to climb out, either by yourself or with professional help. You cannot rest in either of these places. You cannot mend your fabric in either of these places.

Mourning rules from your culture and messages you received as a child are not necessarily bad guidelines for you to follow. Some may be very helpful. Hurting because someone very important to you has died is part of being a human being. Since both death and grief are universal, people at different times and in different communities have learned ways of coping with both loss and pain. All societies have a prescribed way of treating those who die and those who grieve them. These ways of doing things may have continued through the years because they work. They may, however, just be the accumulated junk of the past. You will have to decide if any particular way of doing things or expressing yourself helps or hinders you in your grief.

For example, wakes or visitations can be very comforting if they allow persons to express thoughts and feelings in a safe place, one in which there is neither judgment nor evaluation.

Funerals and memorial services can allow us to move toward accepting that the person is really dead and give us an opportunity to say goodbye. On the other hand, services in which we are expected to act in some way that conflicts with our true feelings may be harmful.

How comforting it would be to be given a single book on how to mend a torn fabric and a list of shops for obtaining the necessary threads and needles. In our society, a bereaved person is given a number of "books" or messages. Often they contradict each other; some have pages missing. As a result, you will have to pick and choose, discard, and begin again. The only true test of whether you have chosen correctly or incorrectly is whether or not something helps you to endure and hopefully move through your pain. If your pain is overwhelming, choosing a way that makes you feel "less worse" than another way may be about all you can accomplish at the time. This is an accomplishment. Do not let anyone, including yourself, take this sense of accomplishment away from you.

There are, then, four paths that may lead you to the places of guilt and/or shame: your cultural background, your personal history, how others define your loss and your response to that loss, and the relationship you had with the person who died. You are probably receiving a number of messages about how you should or should not feel and what you should or should not do. These messages are probably mixed and inconsistent. Some may help you with your mending. Others may disrupt your mending or even cause you to put your mending aside.

If you are grieving, you are very vulnerable. It is easy to fall into or be pushed into a place of guilt or shame when you are in such a vulnerable state. Be on the alert for words that warn you that guilt or shame are nearby: *ought, should, would, could, if only,* and *but.* Denial, anger, sadness, relief, fear, and jealousy are all places in which mending or resting before mending can occur. One or more of these places may even be necessary for certain kinds of mending to take place. You cannot rest in a place of guilt or shame. You cannot mend. Your needles and threads will become so twisted or broken that they are useless. Repeating the following sentences may help you avoid these places.

"Ought," "should," "would," "could," "if only," and "but" are signs that I am near or in a place of guilt and shame.

When I hear any of these words said by someone else, or when I think of them, I will be alert.

I cannot rest in a place of guilt or shame.

I cannot mend my fabric in a place of guilt or shame.

REFERENCE

1. S. Sandarupa, *Life and Death of the Toraja People,* CV. Tiga Taurus, Ujung Pandang, 1984.

Chapter 4

HOW MANY TEARS?

When your fabric was first torn, all you could see was a huge tear in the middle of your material. Perhaps it was so large it was difficult for you to even see your fabric. This may be the way it is for you now. It is possible though that sometimes the tear seems to be different from what it seemed to be at an earlier time. You thought you knew the tear so well and then one day something about it seems to have changed. Your tear, of course, may have changed, perhaps dramatically. The tear in your material may continue to shred. Your tear may also look differently to you depending on what place you are in at any given time. A tear seen from a place of sadness may look quite differently than the same tear viewed from a place of anger. Another possibility, however, is that there is not just one tear in your fabric but rather two or more tears. The tear is not changing. You are looking at a different tear.

Actually, there are always at least two tears in your fabric when someone important in your life dies. There will be one tear in your fabric because the person you loved is no longer physically present in your life. Another tear will be in your fabric because the person *you* were in your relationship with the individual who died has also died. Although this may sound strange at first, think about it for a moment. When a child dies there is a huge tear in the parent's fabric because the child is gone. There is another tear because the child is no longer present for the parent to care for, to nurture, to comfort. Thus, the mother can no longer be a mother to her child, at least not in a physical way. She can no longer do the things for her child that she did as mother when her child was alive. She grieves because her child is gone. She also, however, grieves for who she was as mother to her child. There are two tears in her fabric. One tear is the loss of her child; the other tear is the loss of that part of herself that was mother to this child.

The more important the person who died was to you, the more tears there will be in your fabric. When someone special in your life dies, you may only see one huge tear. Gradually you may become aware of the second tear. Now there seem to be two great ragged holes in your fabric. Important relationships, however, are intricately interwoven into our fabric. If a relationship was very important to you, there will be many tears.

As a father, you may have been the protector, the provider, the disciplinarian and he who threw the ball after supper for your child. Perhaps you coached your child's softball team or soccer team. When your child died, all these different people you were to your child were also ripped out of your fabric. Compared to the enormous tear caused by your child's death, any one of these other tears seems small and insignificant. They may be smaller; they are not insignificant. They do, however, often go unnoticed for a time, then suddenly demand your attention.

Perhaps you experienced a day that was a pretty good day for you. It certainly was not the kind of day you had before your child died. It was not as bad, however, as most or many of your days have been since your child died. Maybe you were able to get some work done; perhaps you even smiled at a joke someone told or even laughed. You came home, ate supper, and sat down to watch television. Suddenly you become very aware that it is 7:30 P.M., Thursday night. This was the time you and your child went to soccer ball practice. Pain sweeps through you as you recall those Thursday nights the two of you would walk together to the practice field. You can almost smell the soccer ball or hear the sound of it hitting the pavement as your child bounces it up and down. This is not the big tear; it is, however, a tear. You cannot be the coach anymore, at least not the coach you once were when you coached your child's team.

People often tell me they feel guilt when they find themselves crying over one of these tears. It seems such an insignificant tear compared to that huge gaping hole in your fabric. It is, however, the particular tear that is causing you so much pain at that moment. It is the tear that requires your attention. It needs mending. Sometimes the big tear cannot be mended until some of these other tears are attended to. Mending these little tears may reinforce your fabric. They may also help you develop mending skills. Allow yourself to focus on the particular tear that commands your attention at the time. Let yourself move from place to place as you contemplate the loss it represents. Stay away from guilt and shame. Just focus on this particular tear in your fabric.

A number of older widows have told me that one of the most difficult times of the day for them is late afternoon. One woman who had been a housewife for over forty years said that she managed fairly well all day until about 5 P.M. At that time she would just "fall apart." Her husband had been dead for some time and she felt she was "getting back on her feet" and then 5 P.M. would come and "wham." I asked her to tell me what she usually did at that time of the day before her husband died. She shared how she would always begin to prepare their evening meal around 5 P.M. It was a time of great anticipation for her. She would think of her day and what she would tell him, and look forward to hearing about his day. She would set the table, perhaps arrange some flowers. "I can't do that anymore," she said. What seemed to bother her the most was that she found this time of the day more difficult than those times of the day or night she and her husband were usually together. She felt she was being very selfish because she was thinking about herself and not about her husband. "It's as though I just want him back so I can fix supper for us again."

Her husband's death was a huge tear in her fabric. Not being able to prepare supper for the two of them was also a tear, however, for she had lost much of who she was when her husband died. The person who prepared dinner for her husband was a very important part of who she was. I suggested that she allow herself to be selfish and to focus on this particular tear in her fabric, to allow her thoughts and feelings to surface, and to honor those thoughts and feelings. She later told me that when she gave herself permission to concentrate on this particular tear, she moved back and forth between anger at her husband for dying and sadness that she could not prepare supper for the two of them ever again. She said that she slipped into the place of shame several times, always when she thought of herself as caring only about herself and not about him. She felt she ought to be thinking about him, not her. The word "ought" warned her, however, and she would refocus on her not being able to prepare dinner for her husband again. As soon as she did this, she moved back into a place of anger or sadness. Eventually she grew tired of working on this particular tear and decided to ask a friend to come to dinner. As she prepared the meal, she cried a little. She also felt good about doing something she enjoyed doing very much.

This is an example of mending/embroidering and we will talk more about this later. It is important now to recognize that this woman could not begin to mend this tear until she allowed herself time in the places of anger and sadness. Her concern with how she ought to feel led her down the path into a place of shame. Sitting in the muck of shame prevented her from doing her mending. It is important that she did not ask her friend to dinner until *she* decided to do so. Asking a friend to dinner because you think or someone else thinks you should do it is not a good reason for doing something. Listen for the should word. It is a sign that you are about to enter or are in a place of guilt or shame. Wait until it is the right time for you.

Many bereaved people have shared with me that they often feel selfish about their grief and this makes them feel even worse. Most of us were warned as children not to be selfish. Perhaps you were even punished as a child for being selfish. The dictionary defines selfish as "devoted to or caring only for oneself; concerned primarily with one's own interests, benefits, welfare, etc., regardless of others" [1]. Focusing on oneself or concern for self, however, is not bad in and of itself. Of course, if we only focused on ourselves and never concerned ourselves with others, the world would be a pretty dreary place. When your fabric is torn, however, you need to focus on yourself. Indeed, except for rest periods when you are in a place of denial, you are forced to focus on yourself. Your loss fills your universe; it is difficult for you to see anyone or anything else. It is also necessary that you spend time focusing on yourself when your fabric is badly torn. How can you mend your fabric if you do not take time to look at it closely? For people who are grieving, however, focusing on the little tears may seem particularly selfish. How can you think about yourself at such a time? You should be thinking about the person who died. Oh my, there is that word "should" again!

Of course you think about the person who died. If your tear is recent, and recent can mean that the death took place within the last few days, weeks, or even months, you rarely think of anything else. When your loved one died though, part of you died also. It is important to recognize all your tears. The big one is obvious. The little tears may not be so noticeable at first. You will become aware of these other tears, however, as the days and weeks and months pass following death. Pay attention to all of the tears in your fabric. You are being selfish, selfish in a good and necessary way. Mending your fabric is the best thing you can do for yourself; it is also the best thing you can do for others. As long as your fabric is so badly ripped with so many tears, just holding your fabric together is about all you can accomplish. Mending even one little tear is an important first step.

Sometimes it is difficult to know which particular tear you are working on. Always start with the pain, not the loss. Follow the pain and it will lead you to the particular loss. What is it that you want right now? What is it that you want to do? Focus on what you want, not on what you or others think you should want. As you do this, the particular loss that is causing you pain at the moment will come into your mind. Of course, you want the person who has died to be alive and with you. That is your big tear. What is it that you want to do with that person at this very minute? You are now looking at the tear that is demanding your attention at the moment. It may be a rather large tear. It may be only a tiny one, especially when compared to others in your fabric. It makes no difference. Stay with the pain.

Perhaps you hurt because you want to go with your loved one to a favorite restaurant again. Allow yourself the right to want to do this. Do not dwell on whether it makes sense to want to do this, or whether or not you have the right to want to do this. Simply focus on what you want to do and allow yourself to move from place to place, thought to thought, feeling to feeling. Stay with this particular tear until you are ready to move on to another one, not because you think you should move on to another. If you honor your thoughts and feelings at any given time, you will move naturally from one tear to another.

Sometimes these additional tears surprise us. We did not realize that some aspect of ourself was that important to us or even important to us at all. It seems inconsistent with how we have thought about ourselves or how we have presented ourselves to others. An example of this is a loss that older adults may encounter when an elderly parent dies. A man in his late fifties told me that he was really puzzled about his reaction to the recent death of his father. His father was quite elderly and had been in poor health for some time. Death was not unexpected. Indeed, both he and his father perceived death as a release from a worn and tired body. This man had seen to it that his father received good and caring attention during his last years and he had also tried to spend time with his father as often as possible. He knew that he had probably not done all that he could have done, but he had accepted that. He was relieved his father's suffering was over; he was also relieved his own responsibility as a son was complete. He was looking forward particularly to having more time to spend with his new grandchild.

Something, however, kept gnawing at him. He said it was as though he had lost something he could not define or recognize. As he spoke about his father, he began to relate things he had done with his father when he was a little boy. As he shared these memories with me, he began to cry. This man was not crying for his father at that moment. He was crying for the little boy who could never be with his father again, at least not on this earth. The man who was crying was a grown man. Even if his father had still been alive, the little boy was only a memory. Yet, in a very real sense, as long as a parent lives, the child lives also. The man looked at me and said, "You would think I was an orphan." I responded, "You are an orphan and you have a right to grieve." I like to share this story in my workshops for it is a beautiful illustration that grief does not have to make sense in the ordinary world.

An old man died; his grown son was now released from his responsibility to care for his aging parent; a boy lost his father.

All three of these events occurred. It was the last of these, however, that caused the man's present pain. This was the tear that demanded his attention. This was the tear that needed mending. It is important to pay attention to these tears for they will not just disappear with time. They require mending. They may require very little mending, but until they are mended, the fabric is fragile. This man discovered that just recognizing the tear, allowing himself to cry, remaining in a place of sadness for a short time, was sufficient. He was now at peace and he left my office eager to begin his new role as grandfather. For this man, the loss of that part of himself as a little boy with his father was a larger tear than the loss of his father. This loss, however, was not immediately recognizable. It could only be identified by acknowledging his pain and allowing his pain to lead him to the particular tear that needed mending at that moment. Before we continue, take a few moments to repeat the following sentences.

When someone important to me dies, there is never just one tear in my fabric.

I have lost the person who died; I have lost part of me also.

All of the tears in my fabric are important; all need mending.

My pain does not have to make sense in the everyday world.

It is my pain, and my pain will lead me to the tear that needs mending now.

REFERENCE

1. *The Random House Dictionary of the English Language* (2nd Edition), Unabridged, Random House, New York, 1987.

Chapter 5

EARLIER TEARS

When someone important in your life dies, there is the tear that results from the loss of that person in your life. There are also the tears that result from the loss of who you were in your relationship to that person. These are all new tears in your fabric and were caused by your loved one's death. There may be tears in your fabric that are not new. They were there before your loved one died. These old tears in your fabric are from old losses, maybe long forgotten. Perhaps these old tears were covered by a temporary patch or held together with some kind of fabric glue. The tear was not mended; it was only hidden. These kinds of tears may remain hidden from view for years. A new tear in the fabric, however, may loosen or dislodge the patch or glue. When the old, forgotten tear is no longer covered up, the pain associated with it will surface. These old tears may demand more attention than the new ones. Sometimes a new tear cannot even be mended until the old tear is taken care of.

There was a woman whose fifteen-year-old son died from leukemia. For the last six months of his life, he had been unable to attend school. His school mates had always been very supportive, welcoming him back to school when he could go, visiting him at home when he was too ill to attend classes. In his final months of illness, at least one came every day to ask about him. They often took turns sitting with him in order to give his mother, a single parent, a little time to take care of chores or even a little time for herself. His death was expected; he and his friends spoke openly about it.

When he died, his friends asked if they could participate in his funeral. They wrote poems, drew pictures, and even decorated his casket. His mother told me that some people may have thought the funeral was strange, but the knowledge of how much these other children loved her child comforted her. She missed her child terribly. She was also relieved that his suffering was over and she sincerely believed that he was in a better place. Her concern was that she could not seem to grieve for him. Her friends told her that perhaps she had done her grieving before he died. Anticipatory grief is possible. She did not think, however, that this was what had happened in her case. She felt that something was keeping her from grieving for her child. As she talked about this, she suddenly remembered a scene from her childhood. A little girl stood in the door watching . . . suddenly the woman began to cry out in a child's voice, "Mommy, Mommy, don't leave me." The memory of that woman's cry remains with me today.

When she was about three years old, her mother had to place her in foster care. Her social worker told her that she should not blame her mother and she should be very grateful to her foster parents for taking her. She wanted to be the good girl that everyone expected her to be; she was afraid of further abandonment if she were not. On the day her mother left her, she waved goodbye, not knowing if she would ever see her again. She never cried. Several years later, her mother returned for her and once again she was warned, this time by her foster parents, to be good and not make her mother feel bad.

Being abandoned by her mother, regardless of the circumstances, was a terrible tear in her fabric, a tear she had hidden beneath a tightly-sewn patch. For over thirty years this tear remained hidden. When her own child died, however, this new tear ripped into a fabric already badly tattered. Every time she even touched the tear left by her child's death, she tore away the patch covering the old tear. The only way she could avoid the old pain, was to deny the new. Only when she allowed her pain to lead her past her new tear was she able to acknowledge her earlier tear. She was then able to sit in places of anger, the anger at her mother for leaving her, and the anger at the social worker and her foster parents for denying her right to feel angry or sad.

As she began to mend these old tears, her fabric became stronger. She was able to return to her son's death and allow the pain associated with this tear to surface.

It is probably impossible for any person to reach adulthood with a pristine fabric. Little nicks go unmended. Larger tears are often hastily mended with crude stitches or hidden beneath the flimsiest of patches. Even with such frail protection or camouflage, however, these tears can often be ignored for years. A new tear in a fabric rips into one of these earlier tears, exposing pain long forgotten or suppressed. Suddenly discovering an old tear may be very frightening for a newly bereaved person; it is easy to fall into guilt or shame. Someone important in your life has just died and all you seem to be able to think about was the time you wanted to go to the circus and your parents took your older sister and her friend and left you at home with a baby sitter. They told you that someday they would take you and perhaps they did, but the memory of being left behind that first time keeps flooding into your mind. It does not make sense. Why do you keep thinking about something so trivial, when you have this huge loss in your life? Actually, it does make sense. A new tear has ripped into an old one. This earlier tear may need to be mended before the new one can be attended to. It is possible that mending this old tear may strengthen your fabric. It is possible that mending the old tear will give you the skills needed to mend the new and more devastating tear. Whatever, it is the old tear that demands your attention. Do not ignore it.

Sometimes these old tears are small; sometimes they are enormous. Sometimes they are tears that have always been acknowledged at least to some degree. Although their presence has long been known, they have never received the careful mending they need. In other instances, these earlier tears have remained hidden for years. It is as though the person has folded his or her fabric over and over to hide these earlier tears both from himself or herself as well as others. The new tear throws the fabric into disarray. Mere handling of the material may pull or snag fragile stitches sewn years earlier, thus revealing the earlier tear. This sudden knowledge of past trauma may be very frightening. There may be flashbacks as bits and pieces of past experience tumble into consciousness.

One man told me that after his son died he began to experience what he described as flickering stills (a series of photographs appearing in his mind). With professional help, he remembered a terrible car accident he had survived as a little child. He knew his father had been killed in an accident; he had not remembered that he had been in the accident as well. If you are experiencing this kind of phenomenon, it is important to realize that this tear has always been in your fabric. It is not a new tear. It will have to be attended to, perhaps even before you can attend to the new tear. Be careful not to fall into a place of guilt or shame. Not remembering does not mean that you are a weak person. It took tremendous strength for you to keep this tear hidden for so long. This same strength will now enable you to mend both this tear and the more recent one.

You may have always known the old tear was there in your fabric, but never fully acknowledged how large a tear it was. A woman came to see me one day concerned that she was not grieving the loss of her mother appropriately. She felt that she should be at least a little sad, but instead she felt frozen inside. She could not explain this. Her life, she said, had been relatively ordinary. Her relationship with her mother had been good. She began to go over some of the events in her life. As she told me about her college years, she calmly mentioned that she had been raped. She had attended a dance, met an attractive young man, and gone with him to his apartment for a nightcap. They were sitting on the sofa talking when he suddenly threw her to the floor and sexually assaulted her. I asked her what that had been like for her and she said that she felt she got what she deserved. She should not have gone with him to his apartment. She told no one.

I reminded her that no one deserves to be raped, regardless of the circumstances. She began to tremble and, in a voice I could barely hear, she whispered that it was the most terrifying and horrible thing that had ever happened to her in her life. She had longed to tell her mother about it, but had not wanted to burden her with the knowledge. She was also afraid her mother would blame her. Unlike the man who had no conscious recollection about his presence at the accident that killed his father, this young woman was quite aware of the rape. She remembered it in detail. What she had suppressed were the feelings associated with this terrible experience. As she began to allow her feelings about the rape to surface, her feelings about her mother's death began to emerge. She moved back and forth, working on one tear at one time, another tear at another time. At times two tears seemed to be connected when she longed for her mother's comfort and support in dealing with the rape. At other times the rape and her mother's death were separate tears.

Sometimes just being in the presence of a person mending his or her torn fabric shines a spotlight on an earlier tear in your own fabric. I have received a number of phone calls from women in their middle years asking me to talk to a daughter, daughter-in-law, or niece who seemed to be having trouble getting over a miscarriage. "It happened a month ago and she is still grieving. She needs to put this aside and get on with her life. Could you talk to her?" I always ask the person who called to come in and invariably I learn that she too had a miscarriage many years ago. It was very early, she tells me. I ask as gently as possible what her baby's name was. Again she tells me it was so early. Her eyes begin to water and she reaches for a tissue, pressing it tightly against her eyes as though to stop the offending flow. I ask again and she whispers that she has never told another person. And then she tells me the name she has kept hidden these many years. She begins to weep freely. At long last she can grieve openly for the baby she lost so long ago. Now she can allow her daughter, her daughter-in-law, or her niece to grieve. This woman's torn fabric is acknowledged and affirmed. She can begin her own mending. She will no longer interfere with the mending of another.

Perhaps someone keeps pulling you away from your mending or calling to you to come out of the place you are in at the moment. Only you can know if you still have mending to do, because only you know if you hurt. If you are in pain, there is a tear in your fabric. If there is a tear in your fabric, you have mending to do. It is very possible that the person or persons who are trying to divert you from your mending have mending of their own to attend. Their own tattered fabrics cry out to them.

Judy Tatelbaum entitled her first book on grief, *The Courage to Grieve* [1]. It does take courage to grieve, an enormous amount of courage. There are often earlier tears to be dealt with. Others may try to dissuade you from your mending, your earlier tears or your more recent ones. They may even accuse you of being selfish, of focusing on yourself too much. Persevere. You will be of little use to others until your fabric is at least partially mended. It is also possible that your persistent labor on your fabric will give others the courage to attend to their own mending. Take a few moments, or longer if you wish, and think about the following.

There may be earlier tears in my fabric.

I do not have to fear these earlier tears.

It took strength to conceal them in the past; this
    same strength will enable me to mend them now.

If my fabric is very tattered, it may take me a long
    time to do my mending.

I will take the time I need.

My mending is a gift to myself.

My mending may also be a gift to others as well.

REFERENCE

1. J. Tatelbaum, *The Courage to Grieve,* Harper and Row, New York, 1980.

Chapter 6

FUTURE TEARS

That single rip into your fabric when the person you loved died was so large and so damaging to your fabric that it was probably some time before you began to notice other tears. Some of those tears were caused by the loss or losses of who *you* were to that person. Some tears were earlier tears that had been in your fabric for years, maybe even since you were a young child. It is possible that the huge tear in your fabric will continue to rip for months, maybe even years following the death. When the original tear keeps ripping, special mending techniques are required. We will talk about tears that continue to rip in a later chapter. There may also be new tears that appear in your fabric weeks, months, or even years, after the person you loved died. These new tears are associated with the original tear, but they are not part of that tear. They represent new losses; they cause new pain.

Professionals who counsel bereaved persons have long recognized a phenomenon referred to as the *anniversary reaction.* Individuals, who seem to be moving through or even past their pain, experience an intensification or renewal of pain on holidays or on days that have a deep personal significance such as the deceased person's birthday, a wedding anniversary, or the day the person died. Sometimes this anniversary reaction is predictable; sometimes it is unexpected. Regardless, the pain can be overwhelming. Understanding the source of these new tears and realizing that this is a new pain may help you to move through the pain without falling into a place of guilt or shame.

It is true that these new tears would not have occurred had the person you loved not died. It is therefore very easy to assume that the new tear is just a further tearing of the original tear. This can be devastating. You have been working on your fabric. It is still frayed, but you have been able to accomplish some mending. You still hurt, but your grief is manageable. The waves of pain still wash over you, but they are not as high as before and the time between them is longer. And then, suddenly out of nowhere, a huge wave sweeps over you, threatening to engulf you. You feel that all the work you have done, all the struggle to pull your fabric back together, or even just to keep it from disintegrating further, is undone. None of your stitches held. It is entirely possible, however, that your stitches have held. Your old tear is not unraveling. There is a new tear in your fabric.

I had heard her story any number of times. She had told me about her fifteen-year-old son, about the night he called to say he would be home in a little while. But he did not come home that night. The police found him in a parking lot. He had shot himself with a gun she kept in the glove compartment. As the months passed, she told me other things about her son. I saw his picture; I came to know him through his mother's memories. This young woman worked diligently at her mending. There were two other children who needed her. Two years passed. Her son was constantly in her thoughts, but some of these thoughts were happy thoughts. The pain continued, but it was manageable. She even experienced some good moments now. She delighted in small pleasures; lunch with a friend, shopping with her daughter, attending a school function with her youngest son.

It was break time at the monthly meeting of Compassionate Friends. She came over to me, a look of concern on her face. I asked her how she was doing, how she was really doing. She said that the past week had been terrible. She seemed to have slipped back to where she was right after her child's death. I asked her if anything was going on in her life that was different in some way. She told me that her son's high school class would be graduating the next week. All of his friends were getting ready for the event. Caps and gowns had been ordered, invitations sent, and plans for the celebration party were taking place. As she talked, I saw a different youngster than the one she had often spoken of before. She was not grieving the loss of her fifteen-year-old son; she was grieving the loss of her high school graduate. This was a new tear in her fabric. It was not as large as the gaping hole left by her son's death, but it was a tear and the new pain was raw and intense.

The death of a child is generally acknowledged to be one of the most, if not the most, devastating losses a person can have. The tear in the fabric threatens to consume the fabric itself. As devastating as this tear is, however, it may be the accompanying and subsequent tears that make mending such a difficult task. So much of a parent's self is invested in a child. As a result there are usually multiple tears around the large gaping one. There is also the likelihood of many future tears since parents tend to mark their lives by the events and accomplishments of their children, whether the children are alive or dead [1, p. 169]. Future tears, however, are not limited to parents whose children have died.

A student came to see me in my office one day. Someone had told her I worked with people in grief and she thought perhaps I could help her. She sat down in the offered chair and I waited for her to speak. She remained silent for a few minutes and then, her voice only a whisper, she told me that she thought she was going crazy. For the past few weeks she had been obsessed with going to her mother's grave. She had been in the habit of going yearly on All Saints Day with her family. This was different. She wanted, indeed had, to go daily. She had trouble sleeping. She had no appetite. She had recently married and her husband was becoming concerned with her behavior.

Her mother had been killed in an automobile accident when she was three years old. No one tried to hide the death from her and she was allowed to cry and to ask questions about her mother. Her aunt and her aunt's husband had reared her as their own child. Pictures of her mother were openly displayed and she was encouraged, but never forced, to talk about her mother as she wished. Despite the tragedy of her mother's death, she had experienced a warm and happy childhood. Going crazy was the only explanation she had for her present state of mind and behavior. I asked her to tell me about her wedding. It was beautiful, she said. Her aunt and uncle had done all they could do to make it a wonderful and memorable occasion. As she spoke, however, she began to weep. There was just one thing missing. Her mother was not there. This was not a three year old crying for her mother. This was a young bride who wanted her mother to be present on such an important occasion. As with the mother whose son would have graduated if he had lived, this was a new tear in her fabric.

Future tears are not limited to events in which the person who died would have participated if he or she had lived. Although your life may seem to stop when someone you love very much dies, it does not. Living people continue to age. As a result, social units may change. If the child who died was the oldest, the age order of the children in that family may remain the same for some time. The family order, then, continues. There is the oldest child who died, a middle child, and a youngest child. When the middle child, however, reaches and passes the age of the child who died, the family order is destroyed. Who is the oldest child now? This is a new loss, a new tear in your fabric. There will be another tear when the youngest child, in turn, also becomes older than the child who died.

People grow older; people move. Moving from one house to another or to another city can result in new tearing. You and the person you loved looked out of a window and saw a tree. This was something you shared. Following his or her death, you continued to look out of that window at that tree. It was a time for remembering. When you move, you can no longer look out of that window and see that tree. Once more, your fabric is torn. It may be only a small tear, but it is a tear. When these new tears are not recognized, they can fray, causing further damage to your fabric.

If the new tear closely follows the original one, it may be hard to differentiate the two. If a long period of time has elapsed, it may be difficult to associate the two tears. Just stay with the pain and honor your thoughts and feelings. Do not get into whether or not you have a right to feel as you do. Follow your pain. It will lead you to your loss.

Some future tears can be anticipated. These tears center around two kinds of occasions. The first are those celebrations that mark events that are commemorated or celebrated by society in general such as Thanksgiving, or Christmas, or Hanukkah. The second are those days that have special significance to you because of the person who died, such as your wedding anniversary, his or her birthday, and the anniversary of his or her death. The tears associated with these two kinds of occasions are often quite different. In the case of those days that are days of general celebration, the presence of others may result in new tears. In the case of those days that have special significance to you, the absence of others may rip into you material.

Bereaved persons often tell me that holidays are particularly trying for them. Not only are they expected to attend family gatherings, they are expected to join in the celebration. This forces them into a quandary. If they insist upon mentioning the person who has died, they risk disapproval from others. This is particularly troublesome if they are chastised, however gently, for making others uncomfortable, for not being able to "get over" the death, or for both. If they pretend that everything is all right, however, they often feel they have betrayed the memory of the person who died. Either way they fail and this failure is a new tear in their fabric.

In contrast, most people, other than the one or two most affected, tend to forget or ignore those days that have special significance because of the person who died. Your loved one's birthday is painful enough. To sit alone and wonder if everyone else has forgotten this person that was so important to you is an additional tear in your fabric. Regardless of the source of the new tear or tears, it is very easy to begin to think of yourself as having slipped back or regressed. You seemed to be doing better. There had been some good days, maybe even good weeks. Now you are back where you started, moving rapidly from one place to another. First anger, then sadness, perhaps fear or jealousy. Huge waves wash over you. Your fabric seemed almost usable again last week; today it appears to be irreparable.

It is important to realize that you are not slipping. This is a new tear in your fabric; this is new pain. You have not regressed. Your earlier work is not unraveling. You do have more work ahead of you because of these new tears. But you are an expert now. You know more about mending than you did before and the tear is not as large. Your high school graduate has died, not your son. The mother of the bride has died, not your mother. Honor your feelings. Follow your pain to the loss. Once you recognize the tear, you will be able to mend it.

If you have new tears in your fabric, it might help to remind yourself of the following.

I have new pain because I have a new tear in my fabric.

I will look for this new tear.

I have survived a tear much larger than this one.

I am skilled at mending tears.

I can mend this one.

REFERENCE

1. T. A. Rando, *Grieving: How To Go On Living When Someone You Love Dies,* D. C. Heath and Company, Lexington, Massachusetts, 1988.

Chapter 7

NEEDLES AND THREADS

No matter how tattered a fabric is, it can be mended to some degree. Some tears may reopen and demand mending again; new tears may appear before old ones are mended. No fabric is torn beyond repair. Every fabric, regardless of its condition, has an inherent beauty. Mending increases that beauty. Your fabric has the potential to be a masterpiece. In order for this to happen, however, you must attend to the tears, rips, and snags that will distort your designs and pictures or perhaps even prevent you from creating new ones. No one else can do your mending for you. You are the only person who can mend your fabric. It will take time, energy, creativity, and courage, especially if your fabric is badly torn. You will have to seek out the needles and threads that you need for your particular fabric as well as for your unique tears. You may have to look in a great many sewing baskets and try out numerous kinds of needles and a variety of threads before you find the ones that work for you. You may find that needles and threads or stitches that worked for you at one point in your mending no longer accomplish what you want to do. You will have to find additional ones to complete your task.

Sometimes you will find encouragement from others, often when and where you least expect it. Other times you may have to resign yourself to mending alone. Relatives and friends may tell you that your tear is not that big or that you should have mended it by now or that it is so large that it cannot be mended. You may be told that certain needles and threads worked well for others; you must not be using them correctly. You may be told that certain needles and threads are unacceptable. People may not want to be around you when you are mending your fabric. It is possible that your mending angers or frightens them because they do not want to acknowledge the tattered state of their own fabrics. And there are always those persons who are convinced they can mend your fabric for you, if you will only do what they tell you to do.

Only you can mend your fabric. Only you can decide how to mend it. Even if you read every book on grief ever written, you may still have to create your own needles and threads or combine several threads to do the work you need to do. You will almost certainly have to use a variety of stitches, possibly on the same tear. You may also find that a stitch that worked at one time for you, does not work at another time or on another tear. The needles and threads described in this chapter, then, are only suggestions. Use, combine, alter, and discard as you wish.

FABRIC CARE

You may be more concerned with your tear or tears than with your fabric. If the tear is a large one, you may not even be aware of your fabric. It is important, however, to pay close attention to your fabric if it is torn. It will need to be handled with care and kept in a safe place. Only the gentlest of soaps or softeners are appropriate. Extreme temperatures or harsh light may cause further tearing. Taking care of your fabric takes time and energy, but it will be well worth it. Proper care of your fabric now will make your work to repair the tears in your fabric much easier.

As mentioned earlier, a physical checkup is an important first step in fabric care. If the death of your loved one was anticipated, you are probably exhausted from the stress of watching this person decline further and further each day in body and possibly in mind. Whether the decline was steady or like a roller coaster, the strain has probably weakened your fabric more than you realize. If the death was not anticipated, the shock of the sudden confrontation with death has stretched your fabric to its limits. Thus, regardless of the type of death, your fabric has been pulled and twisted out of shape.

You may require some type of medication to help you sleep or relax. You do not need medication to help you forget. You do not want to mask your tears or cover them over with a patch. Patches break loose, often tearing your fabric even further. You will have to mend your tears. Medications may strengthen your fabric; they cannot mend your tears. Thus, it is important to find a physician who is willing to acknowledge your tears and your need to mend them, not one who wants to cover them up.

There is also another reason for seeing a physician. It is not uncommon to begin to imagine that you have the same illness that your loved one had. Worrying about similar symptoms will only add a strain to your already taut fabric. Verbalizing this fear, and dismissing it if it is unwarranted, can revitalize your fabric. This is particularly important if there are children involved. I remember one little boy who came to my children's group. His brother died of congenital heart failure. This child was especially disruptive until one night when a pediatrician came to visit us. This kind man drew a picture of what the little boy's brother's heart probably looked like and then listened to the little boy's heart and assured him that his heart was very different from his brother's. The change in this child's behavior was dramatic. Children worry about having the same illness that caused a sibling or parent's death. Adults worry about this also. If you have fears, you are not being silly; you are being human.

Getting a physical checkup is only one aspect of taking care of your fabric. A badly torn fabric needs daily attention. Fortunately you already know what to do. Imagine how you would respond to a call from the hospital. A dear friend is being released and has nowhere to go. You agree to take this person into your home. He or she has had major surgery that removed or damaged large sections of important organs. What would you do for this person? How would you arrange the room? What would you feed the individual? What would you encourage the person to do?

Perhaps a comfortable bed with a lot of soft pillows or soothing music comes to mind; chicken soup might help. Anything you think might help or comfort your friend is what you need to do for yourself right now if your fabric is badly torn. As soon as possible, you might want to encourage your friend to exercise a bit. Maybe just a walk down the hall at first; perhaps a walk down the driveway a few days later. You see, you know what to do to take care of a tattered fabric. So do it, now!

Exercise is important. Your first efforts, however, may be difficult. Grieving uses up an enormous amount of energy. Do not push yourself. A long strenuous walk may leave you exhausted and do more damage than good. Build up slowly. You are not training for the Olympics. You are not engaged in any kind of competition. You are taking care of a tattered piece of material.

What you put into your body is very important at this time. Stay away from alcohol. It may stop your pain momentarily, but alcohol is a depressant. It can only mask your pain; it will not eradicate it. What about smoking? It would be best if you did not smoke. However, you need to weigh the merits of not smoking against the stress of trying to quit when your fabric is already stretched to its limits. This is not a time to prove anything; it is a time to take care of yourself.

Carbonated drinks, highly-seasoned foods, and sugar may place additional strains on a weakened fabric. Plain foods eaten in small quantities throughout the day are probably best. Vitamins may help restore worn places in your fabric. It is best, however, to consult a professional before deciding which vitamins would be best for you to take.

You need exercise and a proper diet. You also need rest. You will continue to need more rest than you needed previously for a long time to come, for grieving uses up energy. Grief work also uses up energy. The desire to sleep more hours at night and/or the need for naps during the day are signs to heed. You want to be careful, however. Naps during the day can prevent your sleeping at night. It may be best for you to rest as needed during the day and sleep at night.

If you have trouble sleeping, you might want to try taking a warm bath before you go to bed, or listening to soothing music. Do not try to force yourself to sleep. Give yourself permission to lie awake. Allow your arm to rest, or your leg. Do not use alcohol or drugs. Use only those medications prescribed for you by a physician who knows your fabric is torn. One physician I know prescribes a sleeping pill to be used only on the third night following two sleepless ones. Be sure to speak with *your* physician before trying this.

Give yourself permission to cry. Avoid the use of so much tissue. When possible allow the watery fluid to flow freely from your eyes and your nose. Daubing at your eyes and nose is a learned behavior that is not helpful. Crying is not a sign of weakness that needs to be hidden. Crying is probably the best fabric conditioner you have available for maintaining your fabric and an excellent needle and thread for mending tears. It is a natural way to release toxins or poisons that have built up; it is a good way to relieve muscular tension caused by stress. It can also prevent further tearing of a ragged rip.

You may not be able to control your crying immediately following a tear in your fabric. Although this may be frightening to you, it is probably fortunate that you cannot control your crying at this time. Later, however, you will become better able to maintain your composure. You may want to do this at certain times or when certain people are near. As soon as possible, give yourself the time and space to cry freely and unimpeded. Do not fear that if you once begin to allow yourself to cry freely you will never stop. You will stop eventually, I promise you. A word of caution for those of you who may not be able to cry. Never force a needle into your fabric. Do not try to force yourself to cry. Accept the place you are in at the moment. Do not let either crying or not crying push you into a place of guilt or shame.

As beneficial as crying is, it does lead to dehydration. You need to replace the liquid that you are losing. Water is the best replacement. Coffee, tea, and carbonated drinks are not good substitutes. Your increased thirst as a result of crying can cause you to drink more of these beverages than you realize. It is a good idea to keep a glass of water close at hand at all times. Place one by your bed at night. You will then naturally consume this liquid rather than reaching for a beverage that may alter your already altered body chemistry.

Crying will probably be especially difficult for you if you are male. I have seen adults tell boy children not yet two years old to stop being a sissy. You may have been told this. It will take a lot of strength and determination on your part to break down this cultural taboo. Do it for yourself; do it for those you love.

Although women are granted more permission to cry than men, they are cautioned to do so quietly. The release of sound is an excellent tool for both fabric care as well as mending. Find a place where you can cry openly. Do not stifle sound. Cry loudly, sob. The more noise, the better.

The need many of us have to hold back or stifle sound is probably one of the greatest impediments to mending a torn fabric. Indeed, repressing sound may further damage your fabric. I am not certain just where the idea of grieving quietly comes from. It is certainly appropriate to scream and yell at a football game. Perhaps grieving quietly is tied to the notion that bearing any pain quietly is somehow heroic. Whatever the source, suppressing sound is damaging to your fabric and detrimental to the mending process.

Screaming may be helpful or even necessary for both release of tension as well as moving through anger. Some people find it easier to scream in the shower, since the sound of the water covers the sound of the screaming to some extent. One man told me that if anyone does hear him screaming in the shower and comments or asks him if he is all right, he just says that he is singing opera. Other people drive out into the country and find a secluded place to scream. Be careful, however, to bring your car to a complete stop before screaming. Do not drive and scream at the same time. You have a right to your feelings. You do not have a right to hurt yourself or someone else.

Some people fear that if they allow themselves to scream, they will never stop. Just as with crying, you will stop. Both are impossible to maintain indefinitely. If you were punished for screaming as a child, you may need professional assistance to relearn how to scream. Effective screaming is a skill. It is worth both time and money to develop this skill. Sobbing and screaming, however, are only two of the sounds associated with grief in humans. Other sounds include keening and toning. Keening is "a lamentation for the dead uttered in a loud wailing voice or sometimes a wordless cry." Toning is a sound that "wordlessly slides up and down the scale, holding an interval, falling off, growing softer, then louder" [1, pp. 142-148]. Another sound associated with grief is grunting which is a guttural animal-like sound.

All of these sounds are natural sounds and in many cultures are encouraged during times of great loss. Although discouraged for the most part in mainline American culture, bereaved persons often tell me about the strange noises they have emitted. These sounds may seem strange to the person who is making them, but they are quite natural. As you become more comfortable with them, you may discover that one is more helpful in fabric care whereas another is more useful when mending.

There are other ways of taking care of your fabric that might work for you. A bubble bath or just soaking in water that is neither too hot nor too cold, but comfortable for you, may help you relax. Some people also find this is a good place to cry. One woman shared with me that she would sit in a tub of water and cry, allowing the water from her eyes to flow freely down her face and into the bath water. She found that letting both the water in her tub and the water from her eyes empty out into the drain was soothing. There was something about all those little wads of tissue everywhere that depressed her. They seemed like silent reminders of her pain. As the water disappeared down the drain, she felt as though that bit of pain was gone. This may not make sense to you. It did not make sense to her either, but it worked for her. If you think it might help, try it; if it does not appeal to you, do not try it. If you do try it and it does not work for you, keep looking.

FABRIC RESTORATION AND MENDING

For some people, massage therapy can be very helpful in restoring a torn fabric, for touch can be very healing. A young widow shared with me that following her husband's death, her massage therapist came to her home. Her therapist set up her table in each room and massaged her as she wept for the life she had shared with her husband in that particular space. She said that some people with whom she had shared this thought it was pretty strange. She, however, said that it was a healing ceremony for her. It certainly did not heal her in the sense that she no longer grieved, but she felt stronger and better able to embark on the mending that lay before her.

Just as with any other professional help, find a massage therapist who will acknowledge the tears in your fabric and your right to mend these tears. If massage therapy is new to you, ask to meet with the therapist to discuss what you can expect and any concerns you may have. This is appropriate and a professionally trained therapist will welcome your questions. You may want to begin with a foot or hand massage, or perhaps your shoulders. What you wear or do not wear is your choice. Some people disrobe for massage; others prefer to remain partially or even completely clothed. Your comfort is what is important. Sometimes when a fabric is torn, touch may be unpleasant or even painful. If this occurs, do not be alarmed. Let your massage therapist know what is happening. What you want and what helps you are your best guidelines, not what someone else thinks would be good for you.

As your energy level slowly begins to increase, you may find that aerobic exercise is useful. Choose the one that is most appealing to you or at least the one that is the least distasteful. You may prefer one that is solitary such as jogging or swimming. You may find that aerobic dancing allows you to be with other people without having to interact to any great degree. Again, do not push yourself. You can stop and rest if you want to. You do not have to keep up with others. Gently ease into a routine. You want to fortify your fabric, not put an additional strain on it. As you become more acclimated to exercise, you may find aerobics a reliable tool for mending purposes. It is a safe way to release anger; it can also provide a closure for time spent in sadness. We will return to this later.

Sadness and anger are two places that many bereaved persons try to avoid, because they define these places as bad places. Neither is bad; both anger and sadness are natural and common responses to loss. In fact, time spent in both of these places is probably essential for the kind of mending that will hold fast through the years. On the other hand, avoiding these places can cause considerable damage to your fabric. It may help you to think of anger and sadness as places to walk or move *through* rather than as places to be *in*.

Few people choose to enter a place of anger. You may not even recognize this place until after you have been there for a time. I have often had bereaved persons come up to me in the funeral home and whisper to me that they are so angry. They cannot believe how angry they are. They are shocked at how angry they are; they may be fearful of being in that place. Being angry is natural. It is what you do with your anger that is important. There are any number of ways of working through your anger. Find one or several that work the best for you. I find jogging, screaming, and gardening helpful.

Jogging, or even brisk walking, is an excellent way to release anger. I picture in my mind the source of my rage and project that picture on the street in front of me. I then stomp on this imagined picture of the person or thing with each step I take. I may combine this with screaming. Always yell *at* the pictured source of your anger; do not just yell about how you feel. Remember that there are no bad words when you are yelling. In fact, you might want to think of the worst word or words you know and then use it or them deliberately. That way you will not spend valuable energy trying not to say something. This can be extremely freeing, especially if one of your fears is that something "bad" might just pop out of your mouth if you let yourself go.

Gardening is another one of my favorite mending tools. I name each weed someone or something that evokes my anger. Then I rip that person or thing out of the ground, stomp on it, and throw it in the trash pile. I not only release my anger in this way, I end up with a beautiful flower bed free of weeds. Some years back a mother who had lost two sons, one in an accident and one from AIDS, came to see me. As we sat in my garden she commented on how peaceful it was. I thought about all the anger I had poured into my garden. Perhaps anger, allowed to pour forth in a safe place, is the best fertilizer for those who wish to harvest peace.

Some people find that physically hitting something is the best release for them. Elisabeth Kübler-Ross and her staff taught thousands of persons throughout the world the art of hitting telephone books with a short rubber hose [2]. Picture in your mind the person that angers you, project that picture onto the phone book, and then pound away. On the other hand, it is possible that your anger may be at something, not some person.

A woman whose husband presumably died at sea in a helicopter crash told me that she was particularly angry at all the forms she had to complete and the hearings she had to attend. She keeps all the papers in a large briefcase and when she finds herself in a place of anger, she hits this briefcase with a child's red plastic bat.

You may want to hit, yet have difficulty engaging in this behavior. Again, do not force yourself to use needles or threads that frighten you or that make you feel uncomfortable. Helen Fitzgerald prepared a list for bereaved children of over twenty things to do instead of hitting someone [3]. Her list is useful for adults as well. Several of my favorites are doing an angry dance, working a wad of clay or play-dough until it is soft, and drawing a picture of what or who is making you mad and then stomping on it.

Others find that breaking something is the best way to release anger. One man shops at garage sales for cheap glassware and dishes. When he finds himself in a place of anger, he takes a box and throws each piece against a brick wall. He then cleans up the pieces and as he said, "get on with my life." If you try this, be sure to protect yourself from flying glass while you are throwing and the broken glass when you are picking up. A bereaved mother told me that she was not comfortable breaking something that another person could use. Instead, she pictures in her mind a china cabinet filled with beautiful crystal. She then envisions herself taking each piece out, one at a time, and throwing it against a brick wall.

Writing is also an excellent way to release anger. Write a letter to the source of your anger. You can write a letter to someone who is living; you can write to someone who is not. You can write to a thought you have or a place or a thing. Write whatever comes to you to write. Pour out your thoughts and your feelings. Remember, however, that this letter is for you. Never, never mail the letter to a person who is still alive. Wanting to mail your letter is a sure sign that you have not finished writing it yet. If your letter is to someone who has died, you might want to burn the letter or bury it in a ceremony of some kind.

In the bereaved sibling's group that I facilitate, all thoughts and all feelings are, of course, acceptable. We have only two rules. You cannot do anything that will hurt yourself; you cannot do anything that will hurt anyone else. Given these rules, it is fascinating to watch each child create his or her own unique way to safely release anger. Some do it with play-dough, some with the puppets. Others hit the bop bag. It is also beautiful to watch the children respect each other. They do not try to change another child's way of releasing anger as long as that anger is not directed at them. They do not interfere with each other's mending. Children have much to teach adults about grief and grief work.

As you release your anger, you may find that you are suddenly in another place. Check for signs that you have fallen into guilt or shame. If not, honor your feelings. Wherever you are is where you need to be at that time. Take a deep breath. It is important to identify where you are. You may have moved to another place; you may have moved to another tear. Take your time. You may find it helpful at times like this to write or draw or work with play-dough. Just write or draw or sculpt whatever comes into your mind. Allow your hands to move as they will. There are several advantages to this technique. First, you release tension. Second, you become more centered. A third advantage is clarification. The particular tear that demands attention at that time may become more obvious. The details of the tear may become clearer.

Acknowledging your anger, affirming your right to be angry, and releasing this anger in an appropriate manner (you are not hurting yourself; you are not hurting someone else) is one of the most effective ways of ridding your fabric of harmful contaminants as well as preparing your tears for mending that will endure for years to come. Hate, however, is not the same thing as anger. Anger is feeling that you have been wronged, that someone or something has been taken away from you, that your rights have been violated. Anger can range from being merely disgruntled to rage. Hate, on the other hand, is quite different. Anger focuses on what has happened to you and what you have lost. Hate centers on the person who caused, or who you believe caused, what happened to you or your loved one. Hate can range from dislike to extreme aversion.

Regardless of the intensity, hate is an acid that is certain to corrode your needles and cause your mending threads to break. Hate that is allowed to fester and grow will destroy your fabric. Getting rid of hatred does not mean that you forgive the person for what was done or not done. It does not mean that you no longer have a right to be angry at that person. Washing hatred out of your fabric is not something you should do for the person who caused your tear or tears. Getting rid of hatred is something you do for yourself. It is not easy to wash hate out of your fabric, and the longer it has been there the harder it is to wash out. You may need professional help or spiritual direction. The first step, however, is to recognize how damaging hate is to your fabric and to permit yourself to want to be rid of it.

The release of anger often moves a person into a place of sadness. After the rage at those who precipitated or did not prevent the tear is released (into the universe, not at the person), the tear or tears become more visible. All that is lost, all that is gone, all that will never be again, is revealed in stark detail. Give yourself permission to sit in this place of sadness. If you will allow yourself time in this place, you will find that it is a place of restoration. Do not let others pull you away. They will try. Just close your eyes, tune them out, and hold your torn fabric close to you. Finger the tears gently; feel the frayed edges. The better you know your tears, the easier it will be for you to mend them. Allow your pain to well up in you. Do not try to push it away or contain it in some way. Welcome it as a part of you and not as some alien thing that threatens to destroy you. Some people find that after a time in this place, they become restless, perhaps bored. Thoughts of new designs or patterns for their fabric attract them. They leave this place, never to return unless future tears call them back. Others find that they need to return to this place, perhaps often at first, and then on special occasions.

If cultural taboos or personal experience make sadness a difficult place for you, the following suggestion may be helpful. Set aside some time to intentionally visit the place of sadness. Decide how long you will remain there. It is always best to begin with a time that is too short rather than too long. I often suggest fifteen minutes at first. Set your alarm clock to signal when your time is up. Allow yourself to enter this place. Allow your pain to accompany you. When the alarm sounds, leave the place of sadness. You can return at a later time. Always plan some activity before you enter the place of sadness. If possible, think of something that gives you pleasure (e.g., bicycling, playing golf, going to a movie, shopping). If that is difficult for you at this time, think of something that will make life better for you or someone else (e.g., clean out the garage, make cookies). Whatever your planned activity, follow through with it when the time you allotted for sadness is ended.

It is possible that you already have all the conditioners you need to care for your fabric and all the needles and threads you need to mend your tears. Think back to your childhood or teen years. What helped you when you were a child and you were angry or afraid or sad? Did it help to have a teddy bear to hold in your arms? Perhaps your old bear is packed away somewhere. Look for it. If not, or if you never had a bear but always wanted one, buy one. Walk through the store and let a bear choose you. No one needs to know that the bear is for you, if you do not want anyone to know. Continue to look in your own sewing basket for forgotten needles and threads. They are often the very best. Be open, however, to new fabric conditioners and new needles and threads. If you remain open, you will find that you have an enormous selection from which to choose.

MENDING PATTERNS OR GUIDELINES

Although books are not necessarily the only or even the best resource for everyone, they may be a good resource for you. I often get phone calls from a relative or friend of a recently bereaved person requesting the name of a book or books that will help. Although these people end the request with the word *help,* I often think they really mean *fix.* This is understandable. The person they care about is in enormous pain. They want to find something or some way to alleviate the pain. There is no magic pill. No book, including this one, is going to restore a torn fabric. Torn fabrics have to be mended. And mending takes time. I usually suggest a book for the relative or friend. That is why there is a special chapter for these people at the end of this book.

You may find it difficult to concentrate on anything for any length of time other than the tear itself. One woman told me that she found books very helpful following her husband's suicide. She threw them down her stairs. It gave her a way to release her anger. Later in her grieving process, however, she found that reading books about grief helped. Although they could not tell her what to expect in the days and months to come, they often helped her to recognize where she had been. She found it comforting to know that others had felt the way she felt.

Be your own guide in choosing which book or books to read. If a book makes sense to you, read it. If not, put it down. It may never be the right book for you. It may be just the help you need at another time. Do not concern yourself with what other people think about a book. Many bereaved persons have told me that Rabbi Kushner's book, *When Bad Things Happen to Good People* [4], was a lifeline for them. One woman told me that she kept a copy of this book in her purse at all times just in case she needed to remind herself of something in it. Just because others find this book comforting, however, does not mean that you will. Do not fall into the place of shame that one man stumbled into. He was convinced that there had to be something wrong with him. The book seemed to help others, but not him. There was nothing wrong with him. The book was just not the right book for him at that time in his life.

If you are looking for a book, you might go to a large book store and just browse the shelves. You can start with the self-help section, but do not limit yourself to these books. One person I know found a book of poetry that turned out to provide just the needle and thread she needed at that time. Another found a biography that enabled her to mend an old tear that had prevented her from working on the new rip in her fabric. For centuries, many bereaved persons have found comfort in the Psalms.

LOOKING FOR
THREADS AND NEEDLES

Some people find that workshops are good markets to look for different kinds of fabric care, new needles and threads, and new ways to use them. Go, listen, and watch the demonstrations; try the new conditioners or needles out if you want to. If not, just think about them. Do not let anyone push you into trying something that does not seem right for you. Take your time. Going to workshops is similar to shopping for anything else. If the salesperson pushes too hard, there is probably something wrong with the merchandise. You are in no rush. Your torn fabric is not going to evaporate. You have the rest of your life to work on it. You never really waste your time by going to a workshop. Even if you do not find what you are looking for, you can at least cross that workshop off as a possible resource.

Support groups are another possible resource. For some people this is a major source of comfort, one that provides the education and training necessary to both care for and mend tattered fabrics. Support groups, however, are not for everyone. One member of a bereaved family may find a group helpful; another member of the same family may not find this to be so.

If you think a support group might help you, look for a group that fits your needs. Support groups for bereaved persons range from those that are run by the participants themselves to those that are conducted by a professional. A particular group may be limited to the original participants or may be open to newcomers. A group may run for a certain number of weeks or it may be ongoing. Some groups invite speakers to address different issues. Other groups are self-contained. The group focus will also vary. Some groups are concerned with grief in general. Others are limited to specific relationships (loss of spouse, parental loss, or sibling loss). Some groups focus on type of death (cancer, homicide).

If the group you are interested in is conducted by a leader, professional or lay, it is a good idea to talk to this person before attending a group session. Find out what will be expected of you; ask, for example, if there is any cost or commitment of time expected from you. If the group is run by the participants, try to speak to one or more before attending. If the group is ongoing, plan to attend at least three meetings before deciding whether or not to continue. Any one meeting can be a disappointment; three meetings will give you a better idea of what the meetings are usually like. Be open to the idea that a particular group may not be for you at this time, but may be helpful at a later date. Some support groups have a list of members who will answer your questions by phone. This may be more helpful to you than the group itself in the early days, or weeks, perhaps even months, after your loss. As with workshops, do not let anyone, family or friends, pressure you into going to a program you do not want to attend.

If there is not a support group in your area that meets your interests and needs, consider starting one yourself. Explore the feasibility with a local church or hospital. There may also be persons attending a local support group who would be interested in forming a group that is more specifically oriented to your needs and theirs. Several parents in my community whose children committed suicide attend the Compassionate Friends meetings for bereaved parents. They also meet with each other once a month as well.

One of the most important functions of a support group is the opportunity to tell your story. You may have had some opportunity to do this immediately following the death of your loved one. Although you will need to tell your story over and over, your relatives and friends may not want to hear it any more. Telling your story, however, is an important part of the mending process. Each time you tell it, the tears in your fabric become a little clearer; the edges become a little more defined. In support groups, you are free to tell your story in exchange for hearing the stories of others. In a real sense, support groups provide an opportunity for you to work on your own mending while learning how others go about doing theirs.

Writing your story can be very beneficial whether or not you have opportunities to tell it. Putting what happened to your loved one and to you, and what is happening to you now, on paper is an excellent way to identify your tears and the places you have been. Keeping a journal can enable you to compare one day or week or month or year with another. You can see what has worked and what has not worked for you. You can see the progress you have made and identify work that needs to be done. As valuable as writing is, telling your story aloud to someone else is just as important. Neither is a substitute for the other. Both are useful and sometimes necessary.

In order to tell your story, you need someone to listen. Sometimes a friend can be a good listener. Explain to your friend that you need a safe place to talk. Ask if you can arrange to meet at a prearranged time. Agree on a set period of time. This is important. Both you and your friend need to set boundaries. Make it clear that you just need to talk; you are not looking for advice or suggestions. You need someone to listen. Perhaps the two of you can arrange to walk with each other daily or weekly. If both of you are careful to adhere to the rules you have agreed upon, this can be a mutually rewarding experience. You can tell your story, the original one or an update, without fear of repercussions or rejection. Your friend can have the joy of being able to do something for you that he or she is actually able to do.

PROFESSIONAL HELP

Writing in your journal, joining a support group, and/or finding a friend who will listen are all excellent mending techniques. It is very possible, however, that at some time in your mending process you will need professional help. This is not because you are too weak to do your own mending. It may be that you do not have some of the needles and threads you need to mend the particular kind of tears you have in your fabric. It may be that your fabric needs special care at this time. It may also be that you need to learn new ways of caring for your fabric or new stitches. If there are earlier tears in your fabric, you may need help in identifying and repairing them. In some instances, you may have to reopen these old tears and remove stitches that have broken or frayed. The best indicator that professional help is warranted is your own feeling that you need help, either because you think, or even hope, that there might be a better way to mend your fabric than the way you are doing it, or simply because you want some help.

Selecting the right professional help is not always easy. There are, however, certain guidelines you can follow. It is important that you go to someone who will acknowledge your torn fabric and affirm your need and your right to mend your tears. You are not mentally ill; you are bereaved. You need someone who is trained and skilled in grief counseling. There are many places to find such a person. A local mental health clinic or hospital might be a place to start. Ask if there is someone on staff who is trained in grief counseling. Steer clear of any agency or clinic that assures you that all of their staff are qualified to do grief counseling. There are many counselors and therapists that I think highly of and recommend to persons who ask me for a referral. Not all of these individuals are good grief counselors. Being a good counselor does not necessarily mean expertise in grief as a particular area.

Your physician may be able to identify an appropriate counselor for you. Many funeral homes now have after-care programs in place and provide information and referral services even if you did not use their burial services. Similarly, a hospice program can often provide information and referral services regardless of whether or not they worked with your loved one. If you are comfortable about doing so, ask friends and relatives who they might recommend. If you are in a support group, other participants may be excellent resources for information on available professional help.

Make a list of four possible candidates. Make an appointment with one of them. If you have bad vibrations (you just do not like him or her) after meeting with this person, try number two on your list. If you do not like this person either, continue down your list. Do not go past four. If you have done your homework, and all four counselors have good credentials and have been recommended to you by others, it is highly likely that you are putting up a block to protect yourself from looking at a part of your fabric with earlier tears or realistically examining some of your stitching techniques. Pick the one out of the four who you disliked the least, and go to this person for at least six visits. Following the sixth visit, reassess the situation. If you still feel that you cannot work with this person, begin the process of looking for someone again.

Professional help need not be costly and may even be free. A number of hospitals and clinics now offer support groups conducted by a qualified professional or a trained volunteer under the supervision of a professional. Some of the best grief counselors I know are priests, sisters, ministers, or rabbis. Look for a person within your own faith network, but do not limit yourself. I have repeatedly had bereaved persons tell me that the greatest source of help for them came from a person affiliated with a religious group quite different from the one to which they belong or in which they grew up. Just make certain that the person is concerned with the tears in your fabric, with your right to mend those tears, and with your right to reject needles and threads that you do not find suitable. Adding members to his or her congregation, or convincing you that some belief is the right belief, should not be one of his or her concerns.

CEREMONIES AND RITUALS

There is a very useful mending tool that is often ignored or minimized in Western society. This is the use of ceremony or ritual. This is unfortunate, because ceremony and ritual can provide a hoop or vise that stabilizes your fabric for both mending and embroidery stitches. It is important in any process, and grief work is a process, to note beginnings, endings, and points along the way that have meaning for the process as a whole. This is what ceremonies and rituals are all about. A ceremony is a planned activity that takes note of or commemorates some meaningful or significant event in your own life or in the life of someone important to you. When a ceremony is repeated through time, it becomes a ritual. Ceremonies and rituals can be personal or collective. They can be private or public. Many societies have a number of ceremonies and rituals that have to do with death and that facilitate grief and grief work, both immediately following the death and for years thereafter. In our society, however, a ceremony for the bereaved is often limited to the funeral.

At its best a funeral allows a bereaved person to celebrate the deceased person's life, to lament the loss of the person in his or her life, and to receive affirmation from others that the loss of that person is a significant loss. All too often, however, the funeral is hastily planned and hurriedly carried out. It is a required performance to be endured rather than an event to be experienced. It signifies an end to grief rather than an important first step in the mending process.

Fortunately for some, the funeral is only the first of many ceremonies that permit celebration and lamentation. Catholicism, both Roman, Anglican, and Eastern Orthodox, provides opportunities for commemorative masses in the weeks, months, or even years following a death. In the Jewish religion, the Kaddish or mourners' prayer permits a public commemoration for immediate family (spouse, children, parents, or siblings) for the first year. Some groups, agencies, or institutions (e.g., hospice programs or hospitals) conduct memorial services although these services are generally limited to membership or other affiliation.

With the exception of the funeral, ceremonies and rituals around loss and grieving may not be part of your cultural or personal background. It is also possible that the ceremonies and rituals in which you have participated have little or no meaning for you or are so emotional that you feel drained for days or weeks afterward. In either case, creating ceremonies and initiating rituals may be an important task for you to undertake in your mending process. If so, there are several things you may want to consider.

A ceremony should mark some event or period that has meaning for the person who lives. It can commemorate or mark an event in the life of the person who died, but it does so because that event has meaning for those who live. The ceremony should provide time to note this event. As with the funeral, there should be opportunity for both lamentation and celebration. A ceremony requires format (i.e., a beginning, a middle, and an end). This format is important, because it provides a vehicle for release of feelings without fear that these emotions will get out of hand. Ceremonies may be personal. They may be social in that two or more participate.

The mark of a good ceremony is the effect it has on the participant. How do you feel immediately following the ceremony? How do you feel the next day, the next week? Do you feel drained of energy? Does your fabric seem more tattered than ever? Are there new tears in your fabric? New tears are an indication that something is wrong with the format or content of the ceremony or that the particular ceremony is not what you need for your mending. If the ceremony is someone else's idea, you can then decide if you want to go to another one of these functions in order to support that person, or if it would be best for you to decline the invitation. This way you can avoid being pushed or falling into a place of guilt or shame. Deciding whether or not to go to the cemetery illustrates this.

For some people, visiting the grave of a loved one is therapeutic. Some find comfort and solace. Others may find this a good place to vent anger or weep. Regardless of the reason, some bereaved persons find they feel better after they have visited the grave of a loved one. In contrast, other people find that visiting the grave leaves them drained or anxious for days following. Family members may differ; bereaved parents may not agree. Respecting your own needs, as well as the needs of others, is crucial.

One bereaved mother told me that going to the cemetery drains her emotionally for days. She goes with her husband two or three times a year, usually on their child's birthday, death anniversary, and All Saints Day. Her husband, on the other hand, goes by the cemetery every morning on his way to work. He only spends a short time at the grave (often drinking his morning cup of coffee), but he says that this is his time with his son. The rest of the day belongs to himself and others. This is an excellent example of a ritual that allows him to contain his grief without ignoring or suppressing it. This couple's child died ten years ago. Both are good parents to their surviving children, productive in their work, and assets to their families and community. On some occasions they do their mending together; for the most part each does his or her mending alone. As he put it, "We just don't go about it the same way. I respect her way and she respects mine."

Revisiting certain places may help you with your mending. The emergency room or the funeral home may provide you an opportunity to work on a tear in your fabric. Plan this event. You may want to call and make an appointment with someone on the staff who will meet with you and answer questions you may have. You might want to ask a friend to accompany you, or perhaps you might ask this person to meet you afterward. One woman told me that she felt that she did not focus at the funeral service for her mother the way she wished she had. She wrote out some prayers and found a poem that had meaning for her. She called the funeral home, made an appointment, and was given a time to sit with no intrusions in the room that had held her mother's casket. She said each prayer, slowly and carefully, and read the poem. She told me that she still grieved the loss of her mother, but now she felt that she had taken care of something that needed to be taken care of. Her fabric still had tears, but one tear was now mended.

Ceremonies often allow us to do things that we thought we had lost the opportunity to do when the one we loved died. A couple in their late thirties came to see me one evening. They had wanted a baby for a long time. At last a child was on the way. A miscarriage at three months left both of them devastated. Yes, they had named their baby. No, they had not shared this name with anyone. There had been no funeral. Family and friends urged them to forget their loss and get on with their lives. As we sat together that night, they both shared their dreams and hopes and wept for all that was lost.

At one point the mother said, "This may not make sense to you, but one of the things that hurts me the most is that I can never buy a birthday cake for my baby." I suggested that she could buy a cake to commemorate what would have been her child's birthday if she wished. She looked up at me, a surprised expression on her face. "I can't buy a cake for a dead person," she said. "Why not?" I asked. I assured her that I had purchased any number of cakes from the local bakery and had never been asked if the person was alive or dead.

Later this woman shared with me an incredible story. She decided to get a cake. Her husband had some misgivings but agreed to participate. The name they had given was inscribed on the cake and on the evening of the day they thought their child would have been born, they lit the candle on the cake and sang happy birthday. It hurt terribly, she said. It was also a very healing time for both of them. She was able to do something she wanted to do. He was able to share that moment with her. The problem was what to do with the cake. They had no wish to eat the cake. Indeed, they did not want to cut into the cake. When we honor our pain, when we work on our mending, we often clear the way for miraculous events to take place. They called a local shelter. An abused child had arrived late in the day and the staff had just discovered that it was the child's birthday. The child's name, you ask? Yes, it was the same name. Again and again I have seen one person's mending bring healing to others. Mending your torn fabric is not an act of selfishness. It is a gift to the universe.

Ceremonies and rituals are excellent needles and threads for use in repairing old tears. They can also prevent new tears from ripping badly. Anniversaries that are anticipated and planned for are often less painful than those that are just allowed to happen. A young man who was a former student of mine called recently to share with me a journey he made to commemorate what would have been his parent's fiftieth wedding anniversary. He was an only child and very close to his parents. Each of their deaths devastated him, but he felt that he had mended his fabric to the point that he could begin to embellish it with new designs. Recently, however, a couple in his extended family celebrated their fiftieth anniversary. It was a gala celebration and he felt cheated both for himself and his parents.

As his parents' anniversary approached, he became more and more depressed. He dreaded the approaching day and wondered how he would manage to get through it. He then decided that he would not let the day control him; he would control the day. He took time from work and flew to the distant city where his parents met and married. On the day of their anniversary, he traced their steps from the room where they met to the church in which they were married. Along the way he encountered people who listened to his story. At first he wanted the day to last forever, but toward the end he knew that it was time to let go. He was tired, but very much at peace. He had celebrated his parents' life together. He paused and then added, "I don't guess I have to tell you that I felt their presence the whole day." He told me that he realized afterward that he had grieved the loss of each of his parents. That day he grieved the loss of his parents as a couple.

Sometimes one ceremony is sufficient to mend a tear or to prevent a tear from tearing even more. Sometimes ceremonies need to be ritualized. One woman told me that the anniversary of her husband's death was a day that was especially difficult for her. The weeks preceding this day were stressful ones as the dread of the approaching day grew. After several years of this, she decided to plan ahead for that day. She gathered together all the cards and notes that she received following his death. On the anniversary itself, she went to his grave and read them aloud. She cried as she read them, but she found it very comforting. This has now become a yearly ritual. It is still a sad day for her, but she no longer dreads it.

VISIONS AND DREAMS

Sometimes fabric conditioners, as well as needles and threads, come to us in extraordinary ways and we discard them because they are presented to us in a way that we do not understand or to which we are not accustomed. They come to us through dreams and visions. I am often asked if I think some experience really happened or if a person in a dream was real. I ask the individual to tell me what he or she felt after the vision or dream. Answers range from "I felt complete"; "I felt that everything was all right"; "I felt at peace."

Honor these feelings. Do not intellectualize them. If you do, you may lose them. You know how you felt. Stay with those feelings. Trust your experience. It is also a good idea to keep these experiences to yourself. You will know when and with whom to share them. Sharing a vision or a dream with anyone and everyone can cause you to lose this gift, because you will focus on the event rather than your experience. Your experience is what is important, not where and when you had the experience. Store your feeling of peace, however brief it may have been, away in your sewing basket. The memory of that peace will provide the brace or backing you need for your fabric while you are mending your tears.

Some people have dreams or visions shortly after the death. For others they may come much later. It is also possible that someone else may have a dream or vision for you. It had been thirteen years since one mother's son was killed [5]. She had been told over and over that, since he was only a child, he was in heaven. Regardless of what others said, she wanted "proof." For several months she prayed that God would send her a message, something that would give her some peace of mind. Although she was a member of a prayer group, she did not share her request with anyone in the group or with anyone else. One day a friend in her group told her that she had something to tell her; she had "seen" her in heaven with a young boy with blond curly hair and blue eyes. Jesus had his arms around the child and Mary stood in the background. As the mother walked toward her child, the little boy said, "Aw, Mom, here you've been worried about me and Jesus gave me his own Mother to look after me." "Aw, Mom," was one of her child's favorite phrases; he had blond curly hair and blue eyes.

The woman who had the vision had never seen this child, neither alive nor in a picture. There was no way she could have known that "Aw, Mom," was how he usually answered his mother. I asked the mother if she regretted that someone else had this vision, not her. She replied that she was, in fact, very grateful that someone else had seen her child. She would have questioned the vision if it had been hers. Was it real or was she just imagining it? Because it was not hers, she could not discard it as something she only imagined. She was at peace; she had received the proof she longed for.

This mother's request for peace of mind came rather quickly. It is important to remember, however, that we do not control dreams and visions. They tend to come when we need them, not necessarily when we want them. A young father wanted a dream so badly following his young son's death. He prayed for a dream; he attended dream workshops. For several years he did everything he could think of to help him dream, but no dream came. He finally gave up. He had all but forgotten his wish for a dream. One night the phone rang. An acquaintance called to tell him about a young couple whose little boy had just died. They were devastated. Could he, would he possibly come speak with them the next day? Of course he would. That night he had his dream. A little boy stood alone. Suddenly his own little son appeared and took the little boy by the hand. Together they walked away, but just as they passed from his view his child turned, smiled, and waved. He had never seen the other little boy in his dream, but he recognized his picture when he went to meet the child's grief-stricken parents. He had seen their child and his in his dream.

MENDED TEARS
THAT TEAR OPEN AGAIN

Some of your attempts to mend your fabric may not work. A young mother's baby died at six months from Sudden Infant Death Syndrome. For months following her child's death, she lived in a gray world. She told me that she had little memory of those months. One day stretched into another; each night seemed an eternity. Family and friends took turns staying with her. Food was prepared by someone and placed in front of her. Just picking up her fork and lifting the food to her mouth was an exhausting task. After a time, however, her family and friends had to return to their own lives. She slowly began to resume those daily tasks expected of her. One task was grocery shopping.

The first time she attempted to shop was a disaster. She had filled her shopping cart, and was even beginning to compliment herself on getting this task done, when she turned to go down the last aisle. She had forgotten this was the aisle with the products for babies. Suddenly she was surrounded by diapers and bottles. Pictures of smiling babies were everywhere. In desperation she fled the store, leaving her filled cart in the aisle. She ran to her car and fell across the seat sobbing. At last, exhausted from her crying, she drove home.

She realized that she would have to do something in order to buy groceries for her family. She carefully devised a plan which enabled her to find all that she needed in the store without ever going down the aisle with the baby products. The night that I shared this story with some bereaved parents, several began to nod knowingly. They knew the rest of the story. One day she entered the store, confident that she could complete this task at least. Things had changed since she had last been there, however. The manager had switched aisles. She turned a corner and found herself in the middle of the baby products. Once more, she fled the store, leaving her basket behind. Grocery shopping for her family was again a traumatic task. A tear she thought was mended had ripped open again.

Mended tears sometimes rip open; new tears appear. Do not become discouraged. Do not let anyone rush you with your mending or push you into a place of guilt or shame. It takes time to find the right needles and threads. The ones mentioned in this chapter are only a few of the possibilities. Try new needles and threads; adapt or modify ones you have used before or that others have shared with you. Discard those that do not work for you. Remember to look in your own sewing basket. Ask people to let you look in their baskets. Shop around (i.e., workshops, lectures, books). If you see something that appeals to you, try it. If not, keep looking. Do not be afraid to try a new stitch. It can be removed if it does not prove to be suitable. Your fabric is much stronger than you probably think it is. It has survived a lot of tears. It will survive your first clumsy attempts to mend it. If you become discouraged, you might want to repeat the following.

It is my torn fabric. I am more familiar with it than anyone else.

It is up to me to mend my fabric; it is my task to decide how to do this.

I do not have to hurry. I can take all the time I need.

I can and probably will make mistakes. I will learn from my mistakes.

Mending my torn fabric is the most important task I have to do.

Mending my fabric is the greatest gift I can give to myself.

Mending my fabric is the greatest gift I can give to others.

REFERENCES

1. D. Feinstein and P. E. Mayo, *Rituals for Living and Dying*, Harper, San Francisco, 1990.
2. E. Kübler-Ross, *Working It Through*, Macmillan, New York, 1982.
3. H. Fitzgerald, *Things to Do Instead of Hitting,* presented as part of the workshop, "Capturing the Interest of Children: Refueling Your Children's Grief Group," fifteenth annual meeting of the Association for Death Education and Counseling, Memphis, Tennessee, April 3, 1993.
4. H. S. Kushner, *When Bad Things Happen to Good People,* Avon Books, New York, 1981.
5. A. Hasling, *Without Neil: The First Thirteen Years of Living with Grief,* 208 Mulberry Drive, Lafayette, Louisiana, 1985.

Chapter 8

COMPLICATED MENDING

The pain of grief is often described as being like waves. At first the waves are huge and overwhelming and the periods between are so short that one wave seems to be immediately followed by another. Gradually over time, the waves become smaller and smaller and the intervening periods of calm become longer and longer. Each loss, however, evokes its own pain. One tear may command your attention at one time; another tear may be more demanding at some other time. Two or more tears may require mending simultaneously. Thus, there may be huge waves of pain from one tear, more moderate waves from a second tear, and still gentler waves from yet another. The more important the person was in your life, the more tattered your fabric will be. Mending a tattered fabric is never a simple task. There is no orderly course to follow. There is no predictable timetable.

Mending any torn fabric requires time and energy, creativity and courage. Some torn fabrics, however, are more difficult to mend than others. They are more likely to require extraordinary needles, unusual blends of threads, and/or a combination of stitches. Although professional guidance may be helpful following any significant loss, it may be necessary if the mending is unusually complicated. Any one of the following five conditions or circumstances can result in tears that are especially difficult to mend. If two or more of these are present, mending becomes even more complicated.

The first factor to consider is the condition of the fabric when the most recent tear occurred. Earlier tears may need to be mended before the new tears can be attended to. In order to do this, however, these earlier tears may first need to be identified. You may have mended earlier tears, but the stitches keep pulling lose. They held for a time and it may be difficult to abandon them for new ones. You may have to do this, however, if you want to mend the new tear. Attending to these earlier tears will require time and energy over and beyond that required to mend the most recent tears. In contrast, perhaps you never needed to mend your fabric before. Thoughts and feelings you have never before experienced may be overwhelming.

A second circumstance or situation that may lead to complications is the potential for future tears. The loss of a child, for example, inevitably results in future tears. A third consideration is the amount of support you will have throughout the mending process. If people are trying to pull you away from your mending or ridiculing you for doing it, your mending will be more complicated. The fourth and fifth considerations have to do with the tears themselves. A sudden and unexpected tear may damage the fabric more than a tear that was anticipated. In addition, unusually traumatic circumstances surrounding the tear (e.g., suicide or homicide) result in further tearing.

CONDITION OF THE FABRIC

Some fabrics were ripped repeatedly before the most recent tear occurred. One of the most tattered cloths I have ever encountered belonged to an older student whose mother had recently died. This woman came to see me because she could not seem to feel anything about her mother's death. She wondered if there was something wrong with her. She asked me if I thought she might be in denial. I asked her to tell me something about her life. Calmly and with little or no expression she told me that she had been sexually abused, as well as physically and emotionally battered, as a child. She had been abandoned and placed in a series of foster homes. She ran away as a young teenager, began to use drugs and alcohol, eventually was arrested, and was sent to a treatment center. She had been drug and alcohol free for several years. She completed her GED (General Educational Development) and had recently entered college. About a year ago, she and her mother had gotten back together. This new relationship was very meaningful to her. Her response to her mother's death was puzzling. "You would think that her death would cause me pain, but I don't feel anything," she said. "What's wrong with me?"

This woman's fabric was so tattered that many of the tears intermixed. At times it was as though only a single frayed thread differentiated one tear from another. I was amazed that she was able to function at all with a fabric in such a tattered state. We talked about her fabric for awhile and I suggested therapy. She asked if I thought she was a weak person. I assured her that, to the contrary, I thought she was a remarkably strong and courageous woman and that she deserved professional help. I recommended a therapist and she called from my office and made an appointment. It was over a year before I saw her again. She stopped by to tell me that she was beginning to feel the pain from the loss of her mother. She had to work on many earlier losses before this could happen. She had a number of tears yet to mend. Even so, the vibrancy of her fabric was already evident. I knew that it would become even more so in the months and years to come.

This woman's mending was complicated because of earlier tears. Sometimes mending is complicated for the opposite reason; there have been no earlier tears. The individual has no sewing basket. Needles and threads were never needed before. The pain from the recent loss may not only hurt; it may be terrifying. Attempts to cope with the terror may cause further damage, even destruction.

A student came by my office one afternoon and asked if he could see me for a few minutes. I was busy and it was not a convenient time, but something about his behavior alerted me. He was a young man and ordinarily full of life; that day he seemed devoid of all energy. He sat there for several minutes and then in a voice I could barely hear said, "I think I am going to kill myself." Suddenly I had all the time in the world.

This young man had lived a storybook life. He had loving and supportive parents and a host of other relatives. He had never lost anything or anyone of value. He had lived in the same house and grown up with the same friends. He had been challenged enough to make his life interesting, but he had never experienced loss. Three weeks before he came to see me, one of his friends was killed in a motorcycle accident. The pain was like nothing he had ever experienced before. It terrified him. We talked for a bit and he agreed to go with me to the university's counseling center. He was placed in the care of a compassionate dorm counselor who continued to reassure him that what he was feeling was natural and that he would survive this terrible pain. This young man was convinced that the pain would kill him eventually; suicide seemed to be his only recourse for relief. Immediate care, compassionate reassurance, and grief education were critical.

Sometimes there have been attempts to mend earlier tears, but the needles and threads were bent or twisted and the stitches did not hold. Even so, the mender was able to keep the pieces of his or her fabric together. These flawed tools and techniques will not work with the new loss. One man shared with me that alcohol had worked for him in the past. When his teenaged son was killed in an automobile accident, however, no amount of alcohol helped. He smiled wryly and said, "I know, because I tried." Alcoholics Anonymous proved to be the best sewing school he could have attended. There he was able to discard his old ways of mending and learn the new stitches that he would need to repair the terrible tears that resulted from his child's death.

Sometimes a fabric is so old, and the tears so extensive, that the owner has neither the time remaining in his or her life nor the energy to mend. Although this is certainly not true for all elderly persons, it may be for some. John and Mary were ninety-two and ninety-four years old respectively. When John died, Mary was content to be John's widow the rest of her life and to live, primarily, with her memories. To ignore her tear, then, was to ignore her fabric. When this kind of tear is acknowledged by others, however, and accepted as the most important feature of the fabric, that fabric can become a meaningful part of a family's heritage. The tear will be treasured along with the beautiful designs and paintings that surround it.

POTENTIAL FOR FUTURE TEARS

The second factor that may complicate the mending process is the potential for future tearing. Mending a fabric torn by a child's death may be a lifetime endeavor. There are so many tears to mend and so many different kinds of tears.

Following the child's death, the family must be redefined. How will the parent respond when asked how many children he or she has? If the parent omits the child, there is a new tear. Indeed, each time a parent leaves that child out, a new tear occurs. Including the child, however, may also result in tearing. People may ask questions; even worse, they may become quiet and look away.

With each advance of the child's friends and/or classmates (e.g., graduations, jobs, weddings, babies) the parent's fabric is torn again and again. On each occasion, the parent grieves for the child "who would have been" had he or she lived. There also will be new tears each time other children in the family advance to a new phase in their lives. This is particularly true when younger children exceed the age of the child who died.

One such family had three children who were eight, five, and two years old respectively when the five year old died. For three years, the parents and the two surviving children thought of the child who died as "the middle child." However, when the youngest child became six years old, this "picture" of the family was shattered. This was a new tear in each of their fabrics. The mother told me that she knew there would always be more tears to mend. When a new one comes, she takes time out to work on her mending. "In between tears," she said, "life is pretty good." It took many years of mending, both the huge rip in her fabric and all the smaller ones, before she reached this point.

SUPPORT FROM OTHERS

The third consideration is the availability and amount of support you will have in the mending process. Mending is complicated when no one will even acknowledge that your fabric is torn, or when your tear is trivialized, or when you are blamed or ridiculed for having the tear in the first place. As mentioned earlier, miscarriages, and stillbirths are often trivialized by family and friends, and chemical pregnancies are routinely ignored by others. It is very difficult to mend your fabric when others deny that there is a tear or tears to be mended. A nun shared with me that following her hysterectomy she wanted to weep for the children she never had. She had not done this, however, since it would imply that her life as a sister was lacking.

A tear that is often hidden from others is a tear from abortion. Even when the tear is known, there is rarely any affirmation of loss. Right-to-life activists question a person's right to grieve when she "killed" her baby. Pro-choice people focus on the right of the mother to choose abortion rather than the emotional consequences. If you hurt, you have a torn fabric. If your fabric is torn, you have a right to grieve. Indeed, if you wish to move through the pain, and you must move through it or it will continue to control your life, you must do your grief work. And that will take enormous courage on your part. If society in general does not recognize your right to grieve, you must demand that right.

There are four aspects of grief work that are especially important when grief is hidden from or disenfranchised by others. These are: 1) claiming the right to grieve, 2) naming the loss, 3) commemorating the loss through ceremony, and 4) sharing the loss with another.

Claiming your right to grieve may be the most difficult for you. You will be told that you have no right to grieve, that your loss really is not as bad as another type of loss, that you should just forget and get on with your life, that you are really fortunate, that it could have been worse, that you are making others uncomfortable. In the case of chemical pregnancy, you may be told that since there was no real pregnancy, you do not have a tear in your fabric. Give yourself permission to respond, to say to these people, "No, you are wrong. I do have a right to grieve because I have lost something very precious to me. I have lost a dream, a hope, a piece of my future. I hurt because I have lost. You may choose not to acknowledge my hurt, but I will not allow you to take my right to hurt away from me."

Name your loss. Speak that name even if when you speak the name, only you hear it spoken. Write a letter to your named baby, crying out your disappointment, your anguish, your anger, your frustration, your sadness. You may decide to put the letter in a baby book, or burn it, or store it in your "grief box."

Find ways to commemorate your loss. One of the most courageous pieces of mending I have ever witnessed was one undertaken by a young woman whose infant son died from multiple birth defects. Shortly after his birth, he was flown to a hospital in a city nearly two hundred miles away. She was not with him when he died. Relatives prevented her from seeing his body at his funeral. One relative told her that she should be glad her baby died because of his defects. Another told her that she should think about how costly her child would have been. No one affirmed her right to grieve. No one wanted to hear her talk about her baby. It was as though her baby never existed. She needed evidence that her baby had existed. At last she went to the hospital where her baby died and literally badgered the pathologist until he loaned her the slides taken at her baby's autopsy. A compassionate photographer copied the best slide and skillfully cleaned and dressed her baby. At long last, she had a remembrance of her baby's life that she could see and hold. It took a long time and the help of others to accomplish this, but it never would have happened if this mother had not first claimed her right to grieve.

If there was no funeral or if you did not attend, plan a ceremony of closure. A ceremony of closure does not mean that you accept the loss, just that you accept that a loss has occurred. The ceremony can be as simple or as elaborate as you wish. You can have candles; you can have music. You can have a traditional ceremony or do something original. Plant a tree, bury the letter or letters that you wrote. You can invite others to attend or you can do this alone.

If you wish, ritualize your ceremony. Select a day, perhaps the day of your initial ceremony, perhaps the day you define as the day your baby died, or the day you think your baby would have been born, or even the day you wish your baby would have been born. You might like to look for a special candle to light. You can do this weekly, monthly, or annually as you wish. Eventually you may want a final ceremony of closure. This is your mending. Do what seems right to you and change or alter what you have done as you wish.

It is important to share both your grief and your grief work with another person. This can be a relative, a friend, a support group member, or a professional. Find someone who can and will acknowledge and affirm your right to grieve. Notice I did not say "understand." No one really understands another person's pain. This is not easy to do, especially if your loss is not generally accepted as a loss in your community. Keep looking until you find someone.

Allow yourself to be creative in your grief work. Since society does not, for the most part, recognize your loss, do not let society direct your grief work. In affirming your pain and thus your loss, you are taking care of yourself. The pain may never go away entirely, but it will become a part of you, not something that controls you. You will also be doing something for others. As you acknowledge your tears and do your mending, you will give permission to others to acknowledge their tears and to begin their mending.

Sometimes a loss is recognized by others, but your right to grieve the loss of this person is not acknowledged. One afternoon my phone rang. I picked up the receiver and said hello. There was only silence for a moment and then I began to hear deep, heart-rending sobs. They continued for some time. I had no idea who was at the other end of the line, so I just periodically assured whomever it was that I was there and would not hang up. Finally, the sobs began to diminish and the person was able to speak. I recognized his voice at once. He was a friend of mine. I knew that his partner had AIDS.

My friend had been taking care of his partner in their apartment. A week earlier, hospitalization became necessary. At that point, the ill man's biological family arrived and asked the hospital to deny any visitors except themselves. They also requested that no information about the patient's health status be given to anyone. This can be done since the biological family is the legally recognized kin if there is no legal marriage or no assigned medical power of attorney. My friend said he would go each day to the hospital and walk by his partner's room. He could not enter the room; he could not learn how this person he loved and had cared for was doing. He told me that he went each day because that was the only thing he could do. The day he called me, he had gone as usual. This time, however, the door was open and the bed stripped of linen. This is how he learned that his partner was dead. His partner's family refused to recognize that he had lost someone very dear to him. He was informed that the police would be called if he tried to come to the funeral.

In a somewhat similar situation, a young woman shared with me that she had been having an affair with a married man who died at his office from a sudden heart attack. She chose not to attend his funeral, for she feared that she would betray their relationship in some way. No one knew about her relationship with this man, so no one offered her condolences. Her pain was overwhelming, yet until she came to see me, she had shared it with no one. She received no permission to grieve. She was beginning to even question her right to grieve. In both instances, finding someone who would acknowledge the loss and affirm the right to grieve was critical if mending was to take place.

Whatever the reason, if grief is disenfranchised, the mending process is complicated. The bereaved person's pain is not affirmed or acknowledged by some other person or persons. The reason the pain is not affirmed or acknowledged, however, is because the loss which prompted the pain is not recognized. The loss may not be known by others, as in the case of the woman who had the affair, it may not be acknowledged, as in the case of my friend, or it may be trivialized, as in the case of the mother of the baby with multiple handicaps. All of these persons hurt. All had torn fabrics. The pain, however, was not validated by others. As a result, all of these individuals were left with a torn fabric and no one to support them while they mended. Indeed, one of them even began to question her right to have a tear in her fabric.

Sometimes the loss is defined as a significant loss, and the relationship between the bereaved person and the person who died is acknowledged, but the loss of that particular relationship is not considered very important. Other people think there should be little or no pain. Again, this is an example of what happens when we start with the tear in order to determine if the pain is justified rather than beginning with the pain.

Friends are often overlooked when a death has occurred. A common expression is that "blood is thicker than water." Relatives are expected to be more affected by a death than friends. The closer the kin tie, the greater the loss. These are mourning guidelines. They belong to the culture and they may or may not describe reality. A friend may be just as devastated as a family member, even more so. Friends are expected to assist the bereaved, however, not be one of them. As a result, a torn fabric may go unnoticed, by the owner as well as others. Again and again, people have told me that they do not think they have ever really allowed themselves to grieve a friend's death. Often it is only when another loss rips into their fabric that the tear from the friend's death is revealed.

Another relationship that is often overlooked is the grandparent-grandchild relationship. When a child dies, attention is focused on the parents. Indeed, the grandparent may be grieving his or her child's torn fabric rather than his or her own cloth. It is only after the parent begins to move through the initial trauma that the grandparent begins to consider his or her own fabric. Since this usually takes a year or more, the grandparent may receive little or no support.

Delayed grief is not always limited to grandparents. Two fathers have told me that their pain was more intense two years after their child's death. In both instances, the father had focused on his wife's loss and pain. Men are expected to be strong and to protect their wives. This is often reinforced by family and friends who ask a man how his wife is doing but never ask him how he is doing. His own tattered cloth goes unattended until her mending is underway. Only then does he turn to his own fabric and focus on his own tears. One man came to me several years following the death of his child. He was concerned because his pain seemed to have intensified. I asked him if it were possible that he had grieved the death of his wife's child for two years and had only recently begun to grieve the death of his child. He paused a moment and then replied, "Yes. No wonder I hurt so much." Delayed grief is always complicated, for none of the usual supports are available at this time. The immediacy is gone and even those who might have been a support have returned to their own lives.

A loss may also be disregarded by others because the particular nature of the relationship is not understood. This may even be true for the bereaved person. The death of a grandparent is considered to be a loss of some consideration, but not comparable to the death of a parent. The grandparent, however, may have been the surrogate parent if the parent was unable or unwilling to play that role. This is not uncommon in families with alcoholism, mental illness, and/or absenteeism whether by choice or not. The person who died may be defined as grandparent of the bereaved person by others, but was, in fact, the person's surrogate parent.

There is one more complication that is probably far more common that most people think. What happens when those you consider to be part of your support system are bereaved persons themselves? When something happens to us that hurts us, we usually look to our family and friends for support. Unfortunately, when a death occurs, our family and friends are often impacted as well. At first glance, this would appear to be a source of comfort. There are two aspects of grief, however, that make this kind of situation difficult for all involved. The first is that no two people ever lose the same person; the second is that each person's grief work is unique.

It may sound strange to you at first that no two people ever lose the same person, but think about it for a moment. A man's wife may die. He is bereaved; his children are bereaved. Each of his children, however, has lost the person who was specifically mother to him or her. Furthermore, the relationship between a parent and a child is influenced by age, birth order, and personality.

When a child dies, both parents are bereaved. But she has lost her child and he has lost his child. To add further complication, she has lost who she was to that child; he has lost who he was. A bereaved mother told me that Saturdays were more likely to be good days, or at least days that were not as bad as others, for her since she spent Saturdays with her daughters while her husband and son went fishing. Saturdays, however, were the worse days for him, for each moment he was reminded of what he and his son would be doing if his child had lived. Each person's fabric is unique. Each person's tears are unique.

Since there is no natural order in the grieving process, each person's grief work is unique. Family members discover that they are often in different places. One may be in a place of denial; another may be in a place of anger. Still another may have completed his or her mending. One bereaved father told me that he dreaded going home on days he felt pretty good more than on his bad days. On his good days, he inevitably arrived home to find that his wife was having a bad day. This would pull him down again. One mother told me that she did not know which was worse, to have a bad day when her husband felt good or to have a good day when her husband felt bad. Because no two people are grieving the same loss and because each person's mending process is unique, additional tearing can take place. You thought this person would always be there for you and he or she is not. This is a tear in your fabric. Or you want to be there for someone and your own grief gets in the way. This is another tear in your fabric, the loss of the person you want to be (e.g., one who helps others). An already tattered material is torn again and again.

SUDDEN DEATH

The fourth and fifth factors that may complicate mending have to do with how your fabric was torn. The death of anyone important to us is always traumatic. When the person has been ill, however, adjustment to the idea of a world without this person can take place bit-by-bit. We have time to say the things we want to say to that person. We have time to say goodbye.

When death is sudden there is the immediate shock of learning that someone you loved is dead. Your body is impacted. You may have trouble breathing; your vision may be affected; your legs may crumple under you. Your mind seems to play tricks on you. Maybe this is only a dream, some kind of nightmare. Surely you will awaken and find that your loved one is really alive and well. And then you realize that you are not dreaming; the person you love is dead. You may continue to go in and out of the place of denial for hours, days, even months following a sudden death. Surely this has not happened, and then you look at your fabric and all you see is this gaping hole. What is happening to you, or did happen to you, is a natural response. Stay away from the places of guilt and shame. This may be especially difficult for you. Indeed, you may need professional help to do this. Get that help.

Each time you exit the place of denial, you want to stop the clock, go back in time, and rearrange events so that the death will not take place. You may play scenes over and over in your mind. What if I had done or not done something differently? What if someone else had done or not done something differently? You want to scream, or wail, or keen. You want to hit something. Trust yourself. Do these things. Just remember that you cannot hurt yourself and you cannot hurt anyone else. You can want to hurt someone. As terrible as such thoughts may seem to you, it is all right to think them. It is what you do with your thoughts that matters.

The rip in your fabric has been so sudden that it will take you days, perhaps weeks or months, even to begin to comprehend the damage to your fabric. You have no energy. Your mind is reeling. You may wonder how others can go about their daily routines when your world has stopped spinning or is spinning out of control. You may get angry at them for being able to do so, or angry at them for trying to push you into doing things you cannot do.

Take your time. Do not rush yourself or allow anyone else to rush you. Your body needs time to heal; your mind needs time to comprehend your loss. It may be months or even longer before you can begin to work on mending your fabric. Taking care of your fabric is the most important thing you can do at this time.

CIRCUMSTANCES SURROUNDING THE DEATH

As devastating as sudden death can be for the survivor, there are circumstances surrounding the death that cause additional tears that further damage your fabric and complicate the mending process. For example, mending will be more complicated if your loved one died as a result of personal carelessness or wrongdoing on his or her part. The greater the likelihood that the death could have been avoided, the more complicated the mending will be. This does not mean that your pain will be greater or lesser than someone else's depending upon the circumstances surrounding the death. It does mean that your mending will be more complicated.

Suicide usually results in a complicated tear or tears. It is very easy to allow yourself to fall into a place of guilt. Perhaps the person tried to call you and you were not at home. Perhaps you were impatient the last time you spoke. People may push you toward this place with insensitive questions about your activities prior to the suicide or your relationship with this person. The behavior of the police may also add stress. The police consider every death a homicide until proven otherwise. This is a matter of protocol. The presence of a note does not change this. All family members and close friends are murder suspects. Each person has to be ruled out. If you are not familiar with police protocol, the sudden awareness that you are being investigated as a possible murderer can be terrifying. Treatment by medics and hospital personnel may have been harsh and impersonal at best, hostile and suspicious at worst.

Members of your family may engage in distorted thinking. There may be efforts to keep the cause of death secret from friends and even other family members. Even when the suicide is not kept secret, reasons for the suicide may be manufactured (e.g., the person knew he or she had a fatal illness). You may become very frustrated or angry with members of your family. You may feel that your friends are too curious or hold you responsible. You may be angry at the person who died for doing this or someone else among your family or friends for not preventing it. You may feel rejected or abandoned. Why did he or she do this without telling you or at least warning you. You may fear your own suicidal thoughts or fear that someone else close to you will kill himself or herself. Suicide results in repeated tears in your fabric, one right after the other, tears that rip into each other and continue to do so, sometimes for years.

If the death resulted from the action of another or others, there are also multiple rips. The person who killed your loved one may not be charged. If charged, he or she may be released. A father whose son was killed told me that the driver who hit his child was intoxicated. He was arrested and charged, but bonded out four hours later. This man was a neighbor and the father had to see him driving down the street almost daily. Each time he saw this man, his fabric ripped again. Even thinking about the person who killed your loved one tears your fabric anew. The intensity of your rage toward this person may frighten you.

This is also true in homicides. You may want to violently destroy the murderer, or even a member of the murderer's family, or you may fear that a member of your family will try to do this. If the perpetrator is unknown to you or not incarcerated, you may fear for your own safety or the safety of other loved ones. The media, the police investigation, and court appearances are all secondary assaults that rip into your already tattered fabric again and again. It is almost impossible to mend this kind of damage alone. Finding help is critical. Indeed, you may have to seek help from a variety of sources (e.g., counseling, participation in several support groups).

As damaging as these types of death are to the bereaved person's fabric, mending some of the tears can eventually take place even if all of the mending is never fully completed. It is difficult to even begin to mend when the body is never found. No matter how certain the death may be, there remains the remote possibility that the person survived. One man shared with me that it made him so angry when the news media kept repeating that his friend was presumed dead following a helicopter crash at sea. He said the word presumed would open up a tiny ray of hope, only to be dashed as soon as he thought realistically about the probability that his friend could survive both the crash and the subsequent days in the water. The original tear was ripped open again and again.

A woman whose husband was missing in action for years said that she just isolated that part of her life from her thoughts in order to keep on going. Keeping a tear or tears contained requires enormous energy and this is containment only. No actual mending can occur. Setting aside a time to focus on your loss or losses and/or spending time with others who have similar losses may help you to place some kind of border stitch around your tear. In time you can even embroider around your tear. The tear remains in your fabric. It will always be there, but it will no longer rip into your new designs.

A single death can be devastating. Multiple deaths shred a fabric almost beyond recognition. This is true if the deaths occur at the same time. It can also occur if one death closely follows another. Each tear produces its own set of feelings that may or may not be consistent with the feelings associated with the other tear or tears. One young woman whose mother died six months after her father was killed told me that it was so difficult for her to mend her fabric. She often wondered which tear she was mending. If she recognized a tear as being one parent's, she felt guilty for not working on the other parent's tear. If she tried to work on two at the same time, her feelings would get confused; she did not know which emotions belonged to which parent. When this happens, it is going to take longer to mend and you may need some special needles and threads.

Death by suicide, homicide, presumed death when the body cannot be found, and multiple deaths result in damage to a person's fabric that requires long and often repeated mending. These fabrics are difficult to mend because the tears are so numerous, so continuous, so intertwined, and so irregular. Attempts to mend one tear often result in further damage to another. One tear impedes efforts to mend another. Just looking at your fabric may plunge you into places so terrifying that your mind seems to splinter into a million pieces. In contrast, a woman whose child was murdered told me that she wished she could go crazy. Maybe then she could forget for a moment what had happened to her little boy.

Regardless whether you feel you are going crazy or wish that you could, you will need support, a lot of support, to even begin to move through the grieving process. You may find that family and friends avoid you after the initial tear. Support groups for persons with similar tears may be the best source of support for you. You may want to join several groups. Professional help is certainly called for and probably necessary.

Do not allow your prolonged need for help to push you toward guilt or shame. The mother of the murdered child told me that she needed so many different kinds of help (e.g., a physician, a counselor, and several support groups). It made her feel that she was a needy person. She was not a needy person in the sense of being a weak person. She needed help from a variety of people because her fabric had been shredded into tiny frayed pieces. No single person or group could help her with all her tears. She needed different kinds of help for different kinds of tears. If your mending is complicated, the following statements may be useful.

If my mending is complicated, I will need help.

Needing help is not a sign of weakness.

I am responsible for finding the help that I need.

Chapter 9

THE MENDED FABRIC

The two questions I hear most often from bereaved persons are: 1) How long will this pain last? and, 2) Will I ever be the same again? The answer to the first question depends on a number of things. The answer to the second question is, no.

The answer to the first question depends upon how torn your fabric was before the most recent death occurred, how many tears the death precipitated, and the potential for further tearing or future tears. A new tear in a fabric heavily damaged from lack of care and/or riddled with earlier tears that were hastily or never mended is more likely to be a ragged rip with frayed edges than a tear in a relatively intact fabric. Attempts to mend the new tear may result in further tearing which may result in an old tear ripping open again. At times these tears may become one, making mending an even more difficult task. The more damaged your fabric was before the death, then, the longer it will probably take you to mend it.

The more important the person was in your life, the more tears there will be in your fabric. You have lost this person; you have also lost who you were in relationship to this person. The more tears, the longer it will take to mend your fabric. It is possible, however, that after these tears are mended, your fabric will stay mended. You may recall this individual with nostalgia, but there may be few if any future tears to contend with. In contrast, you may have sustained a tear that will continue to tear. There may also be a greater likelihood of future tears.

For some people, each wave of pain is followed by a period of relative calm. Then the next wave of pain hits. This process continues but gradually the waves become gentler and gentler and the periods between the waves lengthen. For others the pain never goes away, but if you work on your mending the pain will eventually become a part of you rather than a force that controls your life. For those with extenuating circumstances (i.e., a homicide with all the ensuing investigations and court appearances), grief is like a hurricane. There are periods of intense pain, followed by a period of relative calm until the back side of the hurricane (new court appearances, a newspaper article, a pardon board hearing) hits with a gale force more severe than the previous winds. Your fabric is torn again and again; old tears you thought were mended reopen.

How long will the pain last? It will last until the tears are mended. Will your mending ever be finished? Possibly, possibly not. Each person's fabric is unique. Each tear in a fabric is different. Some tears can be mended so well that there is no more pain. Some may never be mended completely. You will learn to live with these tears; the pain will become a part of you. How long will it take? It will take as long as it takes. You have a right to all the time you need to mend your tears or to make them a part of your fabric. There is no rush. Continue to take care of your fabric. Pay attention to your diet; continue to exercise. Work on the tear in your fabric that is causing you the most pain at the moment.

When pain is so severe it is natural to want to know when it will end or at least subside. This is a time to take care of yourself, to concentrate on getting through each day, a moment at a time. Almost anything that will help you get through a given moment is acceptable. Apply the only two rules that matter. Will it hurt you; will it hurt someone else? If the answer is no to both questions, then do it. No one can take your pain away. It can be masked or hidden, but it is still there. It takes time to mend. It takes work.

Do not let others pull you away from your mending. Do not let others take your needles or threads away from you. Be on the alert for should, ought, and but. One bereaved mother brought a wreath home from her son's funeral. When the flowers wilted, she placed it on her patio. She was not sure just why she was keeping the wreath, but she did not want to discard it. Her neighbor, however, would comment on the wreath every time she came to visit. This neighbor kept telling her that she should get rid of it; it was depressing. I asked the woman if the wreath depressed her and she replied that it did not. She was not certain why, but she wanted to keep it.

I then suggested that she turn the chair that her neighbor sat in away from the window so that she would not see the wreath. The woman later told me that she finally realized why she had kept the wreath. She burned it on the anniversary of her son's death. Trust yourself. I suspect that the wreath depressed the neighbor because of tears in her own fabric. You are responsible for mending your fabric, not the fabrics of your relatives and friends. They will have to mend their own. Do not allow another person's inability or refusal to mend his or her torn fabric interfere with your mending.

I doubt that anyone's mending is ever completely done, especially if the tear or tears were large ones. Old mending gives way; new tears appear. Thus, if we all waited to embroider new designs in our fabric until there was no more mending to do, the world would be a dreary place indeed. It is possible to embellish your fabric even when it is terribly tattered. Someone, maybe even a stranger, may be unexpectedly kind to you. This little kindness may seem like a drop of water on parched lips. It is true that it was given to you by someone else, but you had to be open to receive it. It is only a tiny golden thread among the heavy blacks and brown, but it adds color. The contrast may be startling. Do not rip it out. Take pleasure in it; savor it.

It is possible that you may begin to embroider or paint designs on your fabric without realizing that you are doing so. One woman told me that it had been two years since her husband died. One morning she was working in her garden when she suddenly realized that she was doing so because she wanted to garden, not because it was a way to get through her day. What had been a stitch to hold a tear together was now a stitch with which to embroider. The transition from mending to embroidering is not always this simple. It takes courage to mend; it often takes courage to begin a new design.

It may be that someone or some people are making this transition difficult for you. This may be for a number of reasons.

They may be following some cultural or personal guideline that sets a precise time for grief. I remember my mother telling me that it was not appropriate to use the same flowers for a wedding that were used for the funeral. In other words, a widow was supposed to remain a widow for at least a year following her husband's death. This, of course, is a mourning rule and may have little or no relevance to the presence or absence of tears in a particular person's fabric.

Another or others may want you to focus on your mending because it allows them to ignore their own. There is also the possibility that sitting with you while you mend your fabric has become an important part of who they are. If you stop mending, their fabric will tear. Most people are not aware of what they are doing, much less why they are doing it. You do not need to take on the task of educating them. If you have the slightest desire to try your hand at a bit of painting or embroidering—a class, a trip, a new hair style—do so.

It is possible that your first attempts will be disasters. The butterfly you paint is lopsided or crooked. Your embroidery thread catches in one of your basic mending stitches and loosens it. You attempt a design that is beyond your skill at this time and you have to abandon it. At the very worst, you learn something. It may also turn out that the lopsided butterfly becomes the perfect background for a beautiful flower. Do not force yourself to paint or embroider your fabric. On the other hand, do not be afraid to try. If your fabric needs more mending, you will know. You will hurt. It is that simple. If you hurt, follow the pain. It will lead you to the tear that needs your attention.

Occasionally, a person will continue to mend tears when the tears are apparently mended. There are two possible reasons for doing this. Perhaps you are afraid that if you let go of the pain, you will lose the person you love. Maybe the pain is all that connects you with this person. If this is something you are afraid of, you can relax. The mended tear will always be there in your fabric. Your loved one will always be a part of your life's fabric. You will not forget this person. You may not think about him or her all the time, but you will think about this person from time to time. Your tears are mended; they have not disappeared.

Another reason people continue to mend a mended tear or tears is that they have forgotten how to do anything but mend tears. If your fabric was terribly tattered, you probably have been working on your tears for a very long time. It is possible that you have forgotten how to paint or embroider. Perhaps you never knew how to do this. You have learned how to mend; you can learn how to embroider.

There are several avenues you might want to try. One is, quite literally, to take a course in how to have fun. Courses on how to have fun are often offered free of charge or at a nominal fee. Check local universities or colleges, hospitals, municipal centers, synagogues, or churches. Try something you have never tried before. Break through the cultural barriers. You have probably already broken through several just trying to mend your fabric. Break through a few more. If you are a man, you might consider a course in crocheting; if you are a woman, you might try automobile repair. Do not worry about whether this is the right course for you. You have lived with a terribly torn fabric and survived. You can certainly survive a six-week course.

Another avenue is to reach out and help someone else. This is often suggested as something to do to get your mind off yourself or in order to make you see that there are others worse off than you. Neither is a good reason. Do it as a gift to you. Do it selfishly. Do it because it can provide you with some of the most beautiful threads you have ever seen and you want some beautiful threads in your fabric. Do not take on too much at first. Volunteer to work at a diner for one hour a week or even a month. One man found this especially good for his first attempt at embellishing his fabric. He told me that if one of his tears ripped open unexpectedly and he started crying, he just blamed it on the onions.

A third avenue that is always a good avenue to travel is laughter. Laughter is an excellent tool for mending as well as embroidering. The stitches are usually long-lasting, and the mended tear is often a base for some of the most beautiful designs. Rent some comedies, watch cartoons. Most importantly, laugh at yourself. Make faces in your mirror. The first time or two, you may begin to cry. That is all right. Evidently you needed to cry. Eventually you will be able to make yourself laugh. I have watched bereaved persons move from laughter to weeping and from weeping to laughter. It makes for some very strong mending. It also adds color where before there was only black or grey.

Will your fabric ever be as it was before? Of course not. A mended fabric, no matter how beautifully mended, is never the same as it was in its original state. Perhaps some of your tears will never be mended completely. Your fabric may now be even more susceptible to future tearing. Regardless, your fabric has more potential for beauty than ever before.

When I was a little girl, I was fascinated with the pictures of the medieval tapestries with the unicorns. I loved the beautiful trees with the sunlight filtering through to the ground below. The ground was covered with moss through which peeked tiny flowers in a variety of colors. And almost hidden in the shadows was a unicorn. When I was twelve, my mother took me to New York and there I was able to see a real tapestry. It was even more beautiful than the pictures. Since then, I have always gone to see one of these tapestries whenever possible. Each time I have been filled with joy at the sight of these centuries-old beautiful works of art.

One day I entered a museum and saw that the tapestry on display was at eye level and there was no rope to separate it from the viewer. I was able to go right up to the tapestry. When I did this, however, I was appalled at what I saw. There were numerous tears, some quite large and ragged. Most had been mended in some fashion, but the stitches were often clumsy and the colors were not true. A tear in a blue flower was mended with a blue that did not match and at times even clashed. Even the unicorn looked the worse for wear. I regretted going to that exhibit. I felt that one of the special delights of my life was gone forever. I turned away and headed for the door. Just as I exited I looked back and then it happened. Once more I saw the tapestry in all its beauty. It was vibrant and the little unicorn seemed poised for action. It was then that I realized that it was the centuries of wear, the tears, and the different attempts at mending that provided the depth and texture and vibrancy to the tapestry. A new tapestry might be beautiful to behold. Compared to the old one, however, it would appear shallow and superficial.

No, your fabric will never be the same as it was before. But if you honor your feelings and work on your mending, your torn fabric will provide the background for designs and pictures that were never before possible. Your fabric will become a masterpiece, a treasure for you to own and a gift to all who behold it.

I will honor my feelings and my thoughts.

I will avoid the places of guilt and shame.

I do not have to complete all of my mending to embroider my fabric.

I only have to be ready to resume my mending when I find a new tear or when an old tear needs further attention.

Chapter 10

GUIDELINES FOR THOSE WHO WANT TO HELP

It is very hard to watch someone you care about grieve. You want to do something to relieve the person's pain. You want very much to make life better for him or her. If this grieving person is very important in your life, and if you are honest with yourself, you also want this person to be the person he or she was before the loss. You miss this person in your life. You may be sad; you may be angry; you may be frightened. Read the earlier chapters for they pertain to you as well as to the person you want to help.

Your fabric has been torn by the loss of your friend who now grieves. Perhaps your fabric was also torn by the loss of the person your friend grieves. If your fabric is torn, you may stumble or be pushed into a place of guilt or shame. Perhaps you are being told or are telling yourself that you should put your grief aside. Avoid the places of guilt and shame. You cannot help your friend if you are mired down in the muck of one of these places. You may wonder, however, if you can help your friend regardless of the place you are in. The answer depends on how you define *help*.

If you define *help* as making your friend feel better, then the answer is probably no. You may possibly divert this person for a short time, but the pain is there, and it will be there until his or her fabric is mended. You cannot restore your friend's fabric, because you cannot do the one thing that would remove the tear. You cannot bring the person who died back to life.

You also cannot replace that person in your friend's life. If you try to do this, you will cease to be who you are. That would result in even more tears in your fabric and in your friend's fabric as well. Thus, you cannot "make" your friend feel better; you cannot take away your friend's pain. You can help your friend, however, in several ways.

First, you can help your friend by acknowledging his or her right to grieve. You do this when you listen to your friend even when you have heard the story so many times that you have it memorized. You can also help your friend when you honor the place he or she is in at the moment, regardless of the place and regardless of whether or not being in that place makes sense to you.

Second, you can sit with your friend while he or she mends the tears in his or her fabric. Mending can be a lonely task; it is easier when you have someone to sit with you. The Tiv of Nigeria believe that it is not good to sit alone in the bush [1, pp. 25, 196, 264]. They believe that this is especially so when the person is bereaved. We tend to avoid bereaved persons in our society. Do not abandon your friend. Sit with him or her. You are not there to judge or evaluate either your friend's fabric, or the tears, or the mending. Your presence is what is needed, not your assistance.

Finally, you can walk with your friend. Only two letters differentiate the words "walk" and "work," but these two letters are very important. To work with someone is to try to change him or her in some way. To walk with a person is to accompany him or her. Your friend is on a journey, a journey in search of fabric conditioners, needles, threads, and stitches. You cannot know which or what your friend needs, or when your friend needs one or another. You can, however, accompany your friend on his or her journey to search for them. Before we talk about how you can best accompany your friend, however, review the following basic ideas about grief.

1. Grief is the human response to loss.
2. There is no "right" way to grieve.
3. There is no "right" time frame.
4. All thoughts and feelings are ok.
5. Thoughts and feelings change.
6. We control our behaviors, not our thoughts and feelings.

7. Each person must do his or her own grief work.
8. Given a safe place to grieve, an individual will do the grief work he or she needs to do.

It is important to remember that the greatest gift you can give your friend is the gift of you. It is also important to remember that you are accompanying your friend on his or her journey, not taking him or her on yours. Let your friend lead you. It is his or her loss, not yours. Accept where the person is at any given moment. Allow your friend to concentrate on his or her fabric, or tears, or mending. Accept that he or she may not want to look at the tears, or examine the fabric, or do any mending. Do not push or pull your friend. Walk with your friend or sit beside your friend. Let your friend decide whether to move from one place to another, or to remain in one place for a time.

Immediately following a death, you may be concerned about your friend's physical well-being. Do not offer medications unless you are a physician. If your friend has trouble sleeping, offer to sit with him or her, or be available by phone. Do not worry about whether or not your friend is eating. You can place food near your friend, but do not try to force him or her to eat it.

Do keep a glass of water filled and within reach at all times. If your friend is crying, dehydration may occur. Coffee, sodas, or alcohol will not help your friend. Plain water is best. This is very important, because a person in shock is usually not aware of what he or she is drinking and, because of the dehydration, will drink anything that is offered. A recently bereaved person can mindlessly drink twenty or thirty cups of coffee a day.

Give control to your friend when possible. If he or she is in shock, you may be limited to asking, "May I choose for you?" However, do not take over your friend's life. Remember that you are there to help, not direct. Do not do anything without permission. Do not clean up a room or discard clothes or put away furniture. You may offer to help, or to be present, close at hand, or near a phone. Cleaning up a room, emptying a drawer, or getting rid of clothing are needles and threads for mending. Do not take these away from your friend.

Keep anything and everything your friend tells you in confidence with one exception. If you believe that there is a possibility that your friend is going to hurt himself or herself (suicide), or injure someone else, you need to inform someone with the authority to prevent this from happening. Tell your friend that you are going to do this, or that you have done this, as soon as possible. Keep all other information to yourself. Do not try to serve as a go-between or facilitator unless you are asked to do this by your friend. Even then, ask yourself if you are taking control away from your friend by doing this.

Your friend may talk about the past or future. Feelings are always in the present. Listen for where your friend is at the moment. Do not try to make him or her feel better. Accept where your friend is. Do not say, "You'll feel better tomorrow." You do not know this. Remember that you are there to affirm, not fix. Allow your friend to cry. Do not pat your friend on the head or shoulder; it is condescending. It can also stop a person from crying. Touch can be healing; it can also be a violation to the person. Although hugging can be reassuring and comforting, always ask permission before you hug and allow the person to withdraw when and if he or she wants to.

Do not tell your friend that you understand what he or she is feeling or going through. You do not understand. Even if you have had a similar loss, you only know how you felt. You can tell your friend that you had a loss, but only if it was very similar. Do not elaborate on your loss unless your friend asks you to.

Provide information that you believe might be helpful (e.g., books, support groups). Offer this information three times, then let it drop. Your friend probably heard you even if he or she did not respond, and will ask you about this at a later time if he or she decides it might be a good or useful resource. Do not give advice. A good thing to remember is to avoid any sentence with "should," "could," "ought," or "but."

Do not promise anything you are not certain you can deliver. Do not tell your friend you will always be available. You are a human being and you could be ill, so ill that you are unable to help your friend on a particular day. It is better to say that you will make every effort to get back in touch within twenty-four hours (or whatever is reasonable for you) after his or her call.

Do not offer religious platitudes (e.g., "Your child is now an angel in heaven"). You can say what you believe or hope, although it is best to wait until you are asked. Spend some time finding out what you do believe or hope. Be clear in your own mind before you share with your friend. Do not tell your friend what he or she should believe or hope, or what you wish you could believe or hope. If your friend asks you what you believe, it is always all right to say that you do not know.

Do not try to pull your friend out of a place of guilt or shame. The words "should," "ought," and "need" will only push him or her in deeper. Do not argue with your friend in order to try to make him or her feel better. Do not play a game called, "But you did." Listen. If you must say something, try "That must have been difficult for you" or "You seem to feel bad about that." Remember that you do not have to say anything. Your presence is your real gift to this person, not what you say or do. Do not tell your friend not to think about someone or something or some event. It will only make him or her think about the person or thing or event all the more.

Your friend may get angry with you. If you said or did the wrong thing, apologize. Most of the time, however, it is not what you said or did that evoked the anger. The bereaved person's anger is not directed at you. You are just a safe person. This is a compliment to you. It is important, however, to protect yourself emotionally as well as physically. No one, not even a person with a badly torn fabric, has a right to abuse you, physically or emotionally.

Remember that one of the best ways you may be able to help your friend is to allow him or her to have time to be alone. Perhaps you could take his or her children on an outing or sit with an elderly parent or take care of some chore. Offer no more than three times. If your offer is accepted, make this a priority for you. It is better not to offer anything than to disappoint a bereaved person. Your friend does not need another tear in his or her fabric.

I am often asked if it is all right to cry with a bereaved person. It is certainly all right, but it is important to recognize that you are probably crying because of a tear or tears in your own fabric. Walking with a bereaved person may reveal your own tears. Keep in mind that your friend is the only one who can mend his or her fabric. You are the only one who can mend yours.

Mending a torn fabric takes time, sometimes a very long time. People want to help, but this help is often short lived. There are three things to think about if you really want to help your friend. The first has to do with time; the second has to do with your priorities; and, the third has to do with the state of your fabric.

Time is an important consideration. If you ask a person to give you money for some worthy cause, most individuals will think about how much money they have and how much they can afford to give away. If you ask this same person to contribute time, however, he or she is likely to say, "Sure, count on me." Money can possibly be increased. Time is finite. Decide how much time you realistically can afford to give. It is better to give a grieving person twenty minutes a week consistently for several years than forty hours a week for the first month and then abandon him or her. Once you have decided how much time you can afford to give, stay within this time limit. You will be tempted to give more, especially if your friend's fabric is badly torn or ripped. You cannot mend your friend's fabric, no matter how much time you give. Your friend needs consistent, dependable support now and will probably need it for a long time to come.

Second, get your own priorities straight. I ask each of my volunteer training workshop participants to tell me who is the most important, himself/herself or the bereaved person. The usual answer is, the bereaved person. No! You are the most important person in your own life. You have to be your own first priority. You can only help your friend if you take care of yourself. If you have ever flown, you may remember hearing the steward or stewardess explain that oxygen masks will drop down from above in the event that the oxygen level is lowered during the flight. You were then told, "If you are traveling with a child or person who needs assistance, put on your own mask first and then assist the other person." This is excellent advice for anyone who wants to help a bereaved friend. If you will take care of yourself, you may be able to help your friend. If you do not take care of yourself, you will burn out, abandon your friend, and leave another tear, possibly a large tear, in his or her fabric.

Finally, you need to look at your own fabric. Be honest. Do you have mending you need to do. If so, do it. Do not use your friend's torn fabric as an excuse to avoid work you need to do on your own fabric.

As you walk with your friend, it may help you to keep the following in mind.

I want to help my friend.

I cannot fix him or her; I cannot take away his or her pain.

I can walk with my friend on his or her journey.

This may be a long journey.

If I want to help my friend, I need to take care of myself.

If I ignore my own tears, I cannot help my friend.

If I find tears in my own fabric, I will take time to mend them.

REFERENCE

1. E. S. Bowen, *Return to Laughter,* Harper and Brothers, New York, 1954.

Chapter 11

NOTES FOR THE PROFESSIONAL: THEORETICAL UNDERPINNINGS AND USE OF ANALOGY

This chapter is designed to present and integrate the assertions, concepts, and theories that underlie the analogy of mending a torn fabric. It is intended primarily for the professional who wishes to incorporate the model into his or her work. It may, however, also be useful to those who wish to explore the grieving process at a more academic level.

There is general consensus among both researchers and counselors that a bereaved person has to work through the pain of grief in order to heal. Suppressing or sublimating the pain only delays the work that must be done. The overwhelming pain of grief, however, may paralyze the bereaved person intellectually, rendering him or her incapable of, or at least hindering him or her from, engaging in the essential work that must be done. The need for some kind of direction for the bereaved person has prompted a number of self-help books through the years. Three excellent ones are *The Grief Recovery Handbook: A Step-by-Step Program for Moving Beyond Loss* [1], *Grieving: How To Go On Living When Someone You Love Dies* [2], and *You Don't Have to Suffer: A Handbook for Moving Beyond Life's Crises* [3]. These books offer reassurance that the pain experienced is "normal," and offer practical suggestions for moving through the grief process.

For some bereaved persons, more is required. These persons need a clear picture of the whole grief process; the beginning, the middle, and the end. They need some sort of map which they can pull out and refer to along the journey. They need to be able to see that there is an end to the journey, even though that end is a distant one. The bereaved know what grief feels like. They need to know what grief looks like.

The analogy of mending a torn fabric offers the bereaved person a facsimile of what grief and grief work look like. In so doing, the analogy provides a scenario that contains a beginning and an end, the various components, and the process. It provides a map of the entire journey, or parts of the journey, which can be examined again and again. The analogy of mending a torn fabric also meets certain criteria that are crucial if the analogy is to be used for clinical purposes.

First, the analogy must be both comfortable and comforting. Feelings and thoughts evoked by the analogy itself must be pleasant and positive, never threatening or distressing. Second, the analogy must be familiar, affording readily identifiable concepts with which to work. Third, the analogy must be simple and easily understood. Complex or difficult to understand processes are not only useless to the bereaved person, but may be burdensome as well. Finally, the analogy must be grounded in theory, consistent with recognized and accepted suppositions about grief, and congruent with desired therapeutic goals.

Two examples of analogies that meet most of the above criteria are Bruce Fisher's analogy of climbing a mountain [4] and Richard Kalish's horse on the dining room table [5]. Both are excellent. Fisher's analogy, however, is designed for use following a divorce; Kalish's analogy is useful in understanding a dominant cultural response to death in the United States. The analogy of the torn fabric was designed for bereaved persons following a loss from death. A brief summary of this analogy, the underlying theories and concepts, and suggested uses follows.

BASIC DEFINITIONS

Four concepts are basic to the analogy: bereavement, grief, grief work, and mourning. A bereavement is a loss, any loss. The loss may be a minor one such as losing one's keys, or a major one such as losing one's home or job. Or, the loss may be cataclysmic such as the death of one's child or one's spouse. A bereavement, then, is a tear in one's fabric. Grief is the pain that results from the tear. The use of bereavement as a tear in a person's fabric and grief as a response to that tear are consistent with the way in which both these concepts are used in the literature.

This consensus with respect to both conceptualization and usage does not hold true for "grief work" and "mourning." It is generally accepted that the pain of grief does not just fade away with the passage of time. The bereaved person must do something or at least move through a process in order to adapt or adjust to the loss. Some writers refer to this as "mourning"; other writers use the phrase, "grief work." The roots of this semantic divergence may rest in two quite different intellectual origins.

Rando, a psychologist, writes:

> Traditionally, *mourning* has been defined as the cultural and/or public display of grief through one's behaviors. This definition focuses on mourning as a vehicle for social communication. However, [in her book] the term follows the psychoanalytic tradition of focusing on intrapsychic work, expanding on it by including adaptive behaviors necessitated by the loss of the loved one [6, p. 23].

Thus, Rando uses the term "mourning" to refer to the work, both psychic and behavioral, that an individual must accomplish in order to move through the pain that results from loss.

In contrast, Stephenson, writes:

> The sociological perspective [on grief] differs from the psychological perspective in that it does not emphasize internal feelings. Emile Durkheim, one of the founders of sociology, believed that "mourning is not a natural movement of private feelings wounded by a cruel loss; it is a duty imposed by the group [7, p. 142].

Stephenson uses the term "mourning" to refer specifically to how a person's culture, either internalized or imposed by others, defines loss (bereavement), what the person is permitted or should feel about these losses (grief), and/or what he or she as a bereaved person should or ought to do or not do about the loss (appropriate behavior). He refers to the work, both psychic and behavioral, that the individual must accomplish in order to move toward adaptation or adjustment to the loss as "grief work."

The analogy described in this book is based on a sociological perspective.[1] Culture is too important not to give it a discrete position in the analogy. Thus, "mourning" refers to the way a particular culture defines the tear or tears in an individual's fabric, the appropriate way or ways to respond to the tear(s), and the correct or acceptable way(s) to mend the tear(s). This latter also includes the time that may or should be allotted to the task. "Grief work" is the mending an individual must accomplish in order to repair his or her fabric to the point that painting or embroidering is once more possible.

OUTLINE OF CHAPTERS

Chapter 1

Three theoretical considerations are basic to this analogy. These are: 1) the individual as unique, 2) the individual as a social self, and 3) the premise that an individual responds to his or her definition of a situation, not the situation itself.

The Individual as Unique: Biological,
Psychological, Cultural, and Social Dimensions

When we are born, we are given a piece of fabric. No two people are given the exact same fabric. Even if two fabrics come from the same bolt of material (e.g., brothers and sisters), there are differences, for each piece is cut from a different part of the bolt (gene pool). Each member of a pair of identical twins has a unique fabric. The fabric of one twin may be very similar to the other twin's fabric, but each is unique. They may be genetically identical, but each has his or her own experience. Each one is twin to the other.

---

[1] The conceptualization and use of mourning and grief work does not always correspond with discipline. Charmaz, a sociologist, uses mourning to describe "the process through which grief is faced and ultimately resolved or altered over time" [8, p. 280]. Kastenbaum, a psychologist, uses the term "grief work" to describe this process [9]. Thus, intellectual origin rather than discipline may explain the preference for a particular terminology.

Even if the material is similar, there are differences in dyes. The type of material from which a piece of fabric is cut is also a factor. Some people are given a fabric cut from a sturdy material, one that can withstand repeated abuse. Others may be given a fabric from a material that is fragile and, thus, easily torn.

One person may do very little with his or her fabric, always waiting for tomorrow to come. Another person may actually damage his or her fabric (e.g., substance abuse). Another person may paint or embroider his or her fabric with a variety of patterns and colors, painting or embroidering over previous designs. The treatment of a particular fabric may result from personal choice. Cultural background, however, also affects what a person does with his or her fabric (e.g., whether or not a person embroiders or paints, type of pattern, etc.).

In addition to genetic background, personality factors, and cultural influence, the people with whom a person comes in contact also impact his or her fabric. These people may be caring, abusive, or unconcerned. One may, thus, think of any one individual as a biological entity, a personality, a product of a particular culture, and as a social self.

The Individual as a Social Self

The work of the symbolic interactionists, particularly the work of Charles Horton Cooley who elaborated the concept "social self," is basic to the analogy. The social self "is simply any idea, or system of ideas, drawn from the communicative life, that the mind cherishes as its own" [10, p. 823]. Cooley refers to the process through which this social self emerges as the "looking glass self":

> . . . the social reference takes the form of a somewhat definite imagination of how one's self . . . appears in a particular mind [of another] and the kind of self-feeling one has is determined by the attitude toward this attributed to the other mind [10, p. 824].

In other words, we are not who we think we are; we are not who others think we are; rather, we are who we think others think we are. The social self, then, is as dependent on the group for its

survival as the group is dependent on the continuity of membership for its survival.

Thus, having one's grief affirmed by someone, anyone, is an
important component in grief work. A person is better able,
perhaps able at all, to do grief work when he or she thinks others
think the loss warrants the pain and that the grief work itself
is both justified and appropriate. What happens, then, when
affirmation from others, particularly significant others, is not
forthcoming, or when others, either with or without cultural
backing, define the bereaved person as neurotic or even exploita-
tive? The bereaved person's pain becomes the source of another
tear or tears (e.g., loss of self-esteem, loss of group membership,
loss of identity).

Loss, then, is defined at the personal and individual level; it
is also defined within a culture and by those with whom the
individual interacts. These definitions of loss may not, and often
do not, correspond. In the absence of cultural and/or social support, the pain itself becomes the only affirmation that grief work
is warranted. Throughout the analogy, the bereaved person is
urged to follow the pain to the tear rather than allow the tear, as
defined by culture or others, to justify the pain.

Defining the Situation

At the most fundamental level, a loss is a loss only if and
when what was lost is of value to the individual. Kalish, a
social-psychologist, provides, in essence, a grief theorem: "It
seems fair to say that you can't grieve without being bereaved,
but you can be bereaved and not grieve" [5, p. 182]. Thus, regardless of how one's culture defines a loss or how those with whom
one interacts define a loss, grief is the response to a loss as
defined by the individual.

This view is consistent with the theorem set forth by the
sociologist, W. I. Thomas: "If [people] define situations as real,
they are real in their consequences" [11, p. 475]. The existence
or lack of existence of a tear in a person's fabric is dependent
upon that person's definition of loss. The analogy permits
an individual to define both the existence of a tear as well
as the magnitude of the tear without outside interference or

interpretation. The analogy also provides the possibility of a mended fabric, at least to some degree, and the hope of future worth and usefulness. Further, the analogy encourages the individual to define himself or herself as the only person who can mend his or her own fabric.

Chapter 2

Grief is an experience that can take a number of forms. A person may deny that there is a tear, or if there is one, that the tear is a large one. A person may get angry, feel sad, or feel relieved at the same time or at different times. He or she may get angry at the cause of the tear, at the tear itself, or at his or her own clumsy mending. People even get angry at having to mend. Because of the widespread popularity of the work of Kübler-Ross, these feelings are often referred to as "stages" in the grief process. Since the word "stage" alludes to a series of positions or stations one above the other, I refer to these feelings as places. One can rest in some places, mend in others.

The analogy allows the bereaved person the opportunity to identify where he or she is at a given time (or at least where he or she has been), to accept that place as appropriate without evaluation or judgment, and to move freely back and forth between places. It also encourages the bereaved person to consider how each of these places affects or impacts his or her mending rather than bestowing on these feelings the power to define the worth or merit of the mender. For example, a bereaved person may say, "I am angry so much of the time; there must be something wrong with me." Within the analogy, one is angry because of the tear in his or her fabric. The question becomes, then, "How can being in a place of anger benefit my mending process?"

Chapter 3

Anger, sadness, fear, relief, and jealousy are "natural" emotions in that we do not learn to feel them. True, we may learn how to express them or learn whether or not we may express them. The feelings themselves are attributes of being a human being. In contrast, guilt and shame are feelings that we learn to feel in interaction with others. We cannot feel guilt or shame until we first have learned to think of ourselves in some way. Rando writes: "Very briefly, in guilt the individual perceives her behavior as bad, whereas in shame the individual perceives herself as bad" [6, pp. 478-479]. Either is problematic in grief work at best and "can take on major destructive dimensions" when grief is complicated [6, p. 478]. Guilt and shame, then, are places to avoid or exit.

In order to do this, however, the paths toward these places need to be identified. Four paths, each with its own point of origin, are identified in the analogy: 1) cultural background, 2) personal experience, 3) the expectations of those with whom one interacts, and 4) the relationship one had with the deceased. Once delineated, the individual can then explore each of these paths to determine how or why he or she is in a place of guilt and/or shame with respect to feelings, thoughts, and/or behaviors.

Within any particular culture or among certain people, a particular tear may not be acknowledged or recognized. When this occurs, any attempt to mend a tear may be defined as inappropriate. The grief is disenfranchised [12]. Since only the individual knows how much he or she hurts, only the individual really knows how small or big the tear really is. Understanding the cultural prescriptions, however, can help an individual recognize that his or her grief work may have to be a solitary task.

Chapter 4

The gravity of the loss for the bereaved person is directly correlated with the investment that person had in his or her relationship with the deceased [6, p. 617; 7, p. 125]. Thus, the bereaved person grieves the loss of the one who died. The bereaved person also grieves the loss of his or her own former roles as well as the loss of dreams and expectations. All of these losses need to be recognized. The sheer magnitude of loss when a significant other dies, however, can be overpowering. The analogy of multiple tears in a fabric facilitates the grieving process by allowing an individual to identify the different losses, yet focus on one loss at a time for mending. In essence, the analogy separates the overall goal of mending a torn fabric into smaller, more manageable tasks. In addition, it allows the bereaved person to "normalize" pain that seems to shift or change over time.

Chapter 5

The delineation between "normal" grief and "abnormal" or "pathological" grief is probably one of the least resolved issues in the literature. If grief is "normal," what is "abnormal" grief? Traditionally this differentiation rested on intensity and duration [13]. In the last few decades, this assumption has been questioned.

Is the sudden reappearance of pain always "abnormal"? The concept, "anniversary reaction" suggests that there are extenuating circumstances that "permit" this reappearance of pain. With respect to duration, certain bereavements (e.g., parental loss), or types of bereavements (e.g., sudden death) are now assumed to require a longer grieving process than other bereavements. Regardless, the delineation of normal grief from abnormal or pathological grief continues to plague both researchers and counselors.

The term "complicated grief" has resolved this dilemma to some degree. There is general agreement that certain complications (e.g., ambivalent relationship with the deceased) "complicate" the grieving process. There are other complicating factors as well. These are dealt with more fully in Chapter 8. This chapter addresses one in particular.

Rando refers to "both prior and concurrent losses and stresses" as well as the individual's "mental health" as "mourner liabilities" [6, pp. 454-462]. I like her use of the term "liability." In the analogy, these liabilities are the earlier tears in a person's fabric, tears which must be recognized and mended, often prior to mending the more recent tear. The concept, "earlier tears," allows the individual to assess his or her fabric in a way that does not evoke shame or guilt. It also provides the grief counselor an opportunity to explore with the bereaved person the possibility of rips that need specialized help (e.g., a therapist skilled in childhood sexual trauma) without minimizing the recent loss.

Chapter 6

The reappearance of pain, even intense pain, years after a loss may be a response to a "new" loss which has evoked "new" pain rather than the return of the pain associated with the original loss (death) [14]. Concern with intensity and duration of pain is not limited to researchers and counselors. Bereaved persons are often acutely aware that a sudden reappearance or increase in intensity of pain following a period of relative calm may signal a "failure" in the recovery process. Defining this pain as a response to a "new" loss relieves the bereaved person from the burden of self-blame for regressing and enables him or her to redefine himself or herself as a person who has worked through past grief and can now work through this new grief. He or she is an accomplished mender.

This notion of future tears is especially useful in parental bereavement. As mentioned earlier, the devastation of losing a child is generally recognized in the literature. The individuals within the family are affected, the family as a system is affected, and the passage of time brings further trauma. The analogy allows the bereaved parent to define himself or herself as a skilled mender rather than a failure and to prepare for some of these future tears. For example, will attending a family reunion have greater consequences (and what are the consequences) than not attending it? The individual, then, can choose the best plan (or at least the one that is least worse) for himself or herself rather than be caught off-guard and suffer further tearing [15, 16].

Chapter 7

In order to mend a torn fabric, the owner needs needles and threads. Sometimes these are already available in the person's sewing basket. Sometimes new needles and threads are needed. New stitching techniques may have to be learned. These can be found in a variety of places, but the person will have to look for them and select the ones that suit his or her particular fabric and particular tears. It may be necessary to try quite a few before finding the right ones.

Within the analogy of mending the torn fabric, the individual is presented with a number of ways other bereaved persons have mended their torn fabrics. These are provided as suggestions only. Each individual is encouraged to look for the needles and threads that are most appropriate to his or her fabric and tear(s), to discard those that are not useful, to continue to look for additional ones as needed, and to consider designing new ones.

Chapter 8

The chapter on complicated mending draws heavily on the work of Therese Rando, particularly with respect to her suggested crisis assessment [6, pp. 248-250]. Her five areas of concern and the corresponding depiction in the analogy are presented in Table 1 (next page).

Chapter 9

The length of time needed to mend a fabric depends on several factors. These include the condition of the person's fabric, the size of the tear, the number of tears, the potential for further tearing, future tears, and the type of tear. Basic to the analogy is the notion that there is never just one tear, all tears require mending, mending is work, and mending can only be done by the owner of the fabric.

GRIEF WORK

Although the analogy itself is grounded in a sociological perspective, the basic assumption that a tear requires mending and that this mending can only be accomplished by the bereaved person is consistent with the recognized therapeutic goals of both sociologists and psychologists. Stephenson, a sociologist, refers to three phases in the grieving process: the reaction phase, the disorganization and reorganization phase, and the reorientation and recovery phase [7, pp. 130-141]. Rando, a psychologist, also refers to three phases of grief and mourning: the avoidance

Table 1.

Rando's Crisis Assessment	Corresponding Depiction in the Analogy (the numbers are in the order each appears in the analogy)
1. The nature of the loss and the circumstances around it.	5. The probability that there will be tears that are associated with but separate from the tear that results from the loss of the deceased (e.g., suicide, homicide, multiple deaths, body is never found).
2. Whether the loss was expected or unexpected and the degree of suddenness.	4. A sudden tear.
3. The meaning of the loss and the degree to which it will influence the [individual's] life.	2. Potential for future tears.
4. The [individual's] prior losses and how [he or she] has coped with them.	1. The state of the fabric when the loss occurred (i.e., damaged as a result of earlier tears, a fabric never before torn, previous or present misuse of fabric).
5. The [individual's] current life circumstances and what resources and forms of support are available.	3. Others are trying to pull the individual away from his or her mending in some way.

phase, the confrontation phase, and the accommodation phase [6, pp. 30-43]. For at least two reasons I prefer the "mourning tasks" outlined by William Worden, a psychologist [17]. One is semantic. I prefer the word "task" rather than "phase." The other is Worden's clear delineation between emotional and social tasks.

For Worden, there are four basic tasks: 1) to accept the reality of the loss, 2) to work through the pain of grief, 3) to adjust to an environment in which the deceased is missing, and 4) to emotionally relocate the deceased and move on with life. These are explained more fully below.

Accepting the Reality of the Loss

To even consider the magnitude of the loss of a loved one may evoke such terror that denial is necessary for survival. This is particularly true in a culture in which the word "death" itself is unspeakable (the loved one passed away) and/or talking about the deceased is defined as morbid. Analogies provide a safe place to adjust to an idea or a thought that is too terrible to contemplate in its pure form. The analogy of a torn fabric enables the bereaved person to withdraw from the existential horror without denying the reality of the loss.

Working Through the Pain of Grief

Working through the pain of grief is abstract. How does one work through this pain? What is involved? What is required? For the newly bereaved person, stripped of energy and/or deprived of his or her former source of support, just existing with the pain is difficult enough. The thought of having to "work through it" may require more effort than the person thinks possible at the moment. Again, the analogy provides a picture that "makes sense." It also divides the overall task into smaller more manageable tasks. This is important because succeeding at even one small task empowers the individual to work at others.

This is consistent with Merton's concept of the self-fulfilling prophecy, a natural progression of the Thomas Theorem discussed earlier. Merton writes:

> The self-fulfilling prophecy is, in the beginning, a *false* definition of the situation evoking a new behavior which makes the originally false definition come *true* [11, p. 477].

This is a very useful concept to keep in mind when counseling the bereaved. If the bereaved person thinks he or she cannot mend, he or she probably cannot. Indeed, the bereaved person may create a situation that not only precludes mending but also results in further tears or tearing. Worden writes that, although most people do not take a negative course,

> [Some] people work against themselves by promoting their own helplessness, by not devoting the skills they need to cope, or by withdrawing from the world and not facing up to environmental requirements [17, p. 16].

Mending even one small tear can help the bereaved person to redefine the process as one that is possible rather than impossible.

Adjusting to an Environment in Which the Deceased is Missing

Coming to grips with the full meaning of a life without the person who died takes time. There are numerous little goals that must be reached. For example, a bereaved person may adjust to eating alone, yet be thrown into a panic at the thought of going alone to a movie. Achieved goals may be thwarted. A bereaved person may have adjusted to shopping alone, see a shirt the deceased person would have liked, buy the shirt, and suddenly be confronted with the fact that the person is dead. The analogy allows the person to define these occurrences as new or different tears rather than further ripping of the original one.

Emotionally Relocating the Deceased and Moving On with Life

I have often heard a bereaved parent say that all he or she has left is his or her pain. To give up the pain is to give up the child. Other bereaved persons may also fear that giving up the pain associated with the death of a loved one will result in losing that person forever. The analogy of a mended fabric alleviates the need to hold onto the pain. The mended tear will always exist in the person's fabric. This mended tear may even rip open again. In the meantime, attempts at embroidering or painting can occur. Attempts at embroidering and painting do not negate the relationship between the bereaved person and his or her loved one.

The analogy of mending a torn fabric, then, meets the outlined criteria. First, it is comfortable and comforting. Needlework is usually associated with motherly or grandmotherly activities, evoking warm and positive feelings. Second, it presents a familiar picture. Even if the person is not skilled or experienced in the art of mending, concepts such as needles and threads, fabric conditioners, and stitches are readily recognized. Third, the analogy is simple. The total scenario is easily grasped and the parts of it make sense in and of themselves. This is especially important for bereaved persons who may have difficulty focusing on any one part or even holding a train of thought for any period of time. Finally, the analogy is consistent with accepted suppositions about grief, is grounded in theory, and is congruent with recognized therapeutic goals.

The uniqueness of the individual is inherent in the analogy. Genetic factors, the impact of culture, and the influence of past personal experience are considered. The concepts of role, role reciprocity, the social self, and the meaning an individual attributes to self and others are integrated components. Finally, the analogy presents a realistic goal. The individual will not return to the person he or she was before the death. His or her fabric will never be as it was before the loss. On the other hand, a mended fabric is a realistic possibility. Further, the image of a mended fabric holds out the possibility of new designs, yet does not mandate the denial of the former relationship.

Change is inherent in both the tearing and mending processes. Although change may necessitate finding new ways to mend, it is not defined as destructive. The analogy provides a vehicle through which an individual is empowered to be self-directed, yet able to look for and receive assistance from others. The bereaved person can employ skills learned through past experience as well as through observation of others. He or she can discard ineffective or damaging tools (e.g., beliefs and behaviors). The analogy challenges the individual to be creative rather than competitive. It presents a realistic goal, continued growth, rather than a fantasy of returning to a former more perfect or at least less blemished self.

SUGGESTIONS FOR USING
THE ANALOGY

Society (those not directly affected by a death) tends to focus on the loss. A bereaved person who seeks counseling is focused on the pain. This may be shortly after a death has occurred; it can be much later in the process. This makes sense, since it is the pain that drives an individual to seek help. The pain, itself, is terrifying. Is it "normal" to hurt so much? Will it ever stop? Am I going crazy? Am I already crazy?

In the early period of grief, I often use a piece of fabric with multiple tears in it to help the person "see" what is happening. Later, I may use this visual aid to help the person identify additional tears associated with the loss of the loved one, earlier tears that may complicate mending, and tears that may be subsequent to the loss (future tears). I have also used this visual aid to help family or friends comprehend what the bereaved person is going through, particularly when the grief is complicated.

Because sewing is universally recognized, the analogy provides a commonality for persons with different life experiences, both cultural and personal. Thus, it can be used when the counselor and client have different life styles or class differences. It can also be useful in groups when the group participants have little in common with each other. In each of these instances, the analogy becomes a meeting place for those involved.

Since the analogy can be presented verbally or visually through a torn piece of material, it is also useful for different age and educational levels (e.g., persons in the same family or in the same community). It also can be used with the mentally challenged individual or when verbal communication is minimal.

The analogy can be presented to the bereaved individual in its entirety or apportioned by chapter. The analogy is useful for crisis intervention, one-time workshops, or groups of longer duration. I have also found it to be useful in training persons who will come in contact with the bereaved (e.g., hospice volunteers).

The needles and threads, the stitching techniques, and the patterns are presented in the analogy as suggestions, not directions. The reader is encouraged to use, combine, alter, and discard as he or she wishes. The same holds true for the grief counselor or therapist [17]. Feel free to use the analogy in new ways, or to develop the analogy to fit your particular practice. If you do this, however, it is important for you to continue to test the linkage between your use of the analogy and both recognized suppositions about grief and your desired therapeutic goal. Finally, remember to take care of yourself. It is difficult to assist others with their mending when our own fabric cries out for attention.

REFERENCES

1. J. James and F. Cherry, *The Grief Recovery Handbook: A Step-by-Step Program for Moving Beyond Loss,* Harper and Row, New York, 1988.
2. T. A. Rando, *Grieving: How To Go On Living When Someone You Love Dies,* Lexington Books, Lexington, Massachusetts, 1988.
3. J. Tatelbaum, *You Don't Have to Suffer: A Handbook for Moving Beyond Life's Crises,* Harper & Row Publishers, New York, 1989.
4. B. Fisher, *Rebuilding: When Your Relationship Ends,* Impact Publishers, San Luis Obispo, California, 1981.
5. R. Kalish, *Death, Grief, and Caring Relationships,* Brooks/Cole, Monterey, California, 1985.
6. T. A. Rando, *Treatment of Complicated Mourning,* Research Press, Champaign, Illinois, 1993.
7. J. S. Stephenson, *Death, Grief, and Mourning: Individual and Social Realities,* The Free Press, New York, 1985.
8. K. Charmaz, *The Social Reality of Death,* Addison-Wesley, Menlo Park, California, 1980.
9. R. J. Kastenbaum, *Death, Society, and Human Experience,* Allyn & Bacon, Needham Heights, Massachusetts, 1995.
10. C. H. Cooley, The Social Self, in *Theories of Society,* T. Parsons et al. (eds.), The Free Press, New York, pp. 822-828, 1961.
11. R. K. Merton, *Social Theory and Social Structure,* The Free Press, New York, 1968.
12. K. J. Doka (ed.), *Disenfranchised Grief: Recognizing Hidden Sorrow,* Lexington, Lexington, Massachusetts, 1989.
13. S. Freud, Mourning and Melancholia, in *The Complete Psychological Works of Sigmund Freud,* J. Strachey (trans.), The Hogarth Press, London, pp. 243-257, 1957.

14. S. Brabant, Old Pain or New Pain: A Social Psychological Approach to Recurrent Grief, *Omega, 20*:4, pp. 273-279, 1989-90.
15. S. Brabant, C. Forsyth, and G. McFarlain, Defining the Family After the Death of a Child, *Death Studies, 18*:2, pp. 197-206, 1994.
16. S. Brabant, C. Forsyth, and G. McFarlain, Special Moments, Special Times: Problematic Occasions Following the Death of a Child, *Clinical Sociology Review 13,* pp. 57-69, 1995.
17. J. W. Worden, *Grief Counseling and Grief Therapy,* Springer Publishing Company, New York, 1991.

BIBLIOGRAPHY

Brabant, S., Old Pain or New Pain: A Social Psychological Approach to Recurrent Grief, *Omega, 20*:4, pp. 273-279, 1989-90.

Brabant, S., C. Forsyth, and G. McFarlain, Defining the Family After the Death of a Child, *Death Studies, 18*:2, pp. 197-206, 1994.

Brabant, S., C. Forsyth, and G. McFarlain, Special Moments, Special Times: Problematic Occasions Following the Death of a Child, *Clinical Sociology Review, 13,* pp. 57-69, 1995.

Bowen, E. S., *Return to Laughter,* Harper and Brothers, New York, 1954.

Cooley, C. H., The Social Self, in *Theories of Society,* T. Parsons et al. (eds.), The Free Press, New York, pp. 822-828, 1961.

Doka, K. J. (ed.), *Disenfranchised Grief: Recognizing Hidden Sorrow,* Lexington, Lexington, Massachusetts, 1989.

Feinstein, D. and P. E. Mayo, *Rituals for Living and Dying,* Harper, San Francisco, 1990.

Fisher, B., *Rebuilding: When Your Relationship Ends,* Impact Publishers, San Luis Obispo, California, 1981.

Fitzgerald, H., *Things to Do Instead of Hitting,* presented as part of the workshop, "Capturing the Interest of Children: Refueling Your Children's Grief Group," fifteenth annual meeting of the Association for Death Education and Counseling, Memphis, Tennessee, April 3, 1993.

Freud, S., Mourning and Melancholia, in *The Complete Psychological Works of Sigmund Freud,* J. Strachey (trans.), The Hogarth Press, London, pp. 243-257, 1957.

Hasling, A., *Without Neil: The First Thirteen Years of Living with Grief,* 208 Mulberry Drive, Lafayette, Louisiana, 1985.

James, J. and F. Cherry, *The Grief Recovery Handbook: A Step-by-Step Program for Moving Beyond Loss,* Harper and Row, New York, 1988.

145

Kalish, R., *Death, Grief, and Caring Relationships,* Brooks/Cole, Monterey, California, 1985.

Kübler-Ross, E., *On Death and Dying,* Preface, Macmillan, New York, 1967.

Kübler-Ross, E., *Working It Through,* Macmillan, New York, 1982.

Kushner, H. S., *When Bad Things Happen to Good People,* Avon Books, New York, 1981.

Langford, M., *That Nothing Be Wasted,* New Hope, Birmingham, Alabama, 1988.

Levoy, G., Tears That Speak, *Psychology Today, 22:*7/8, pp. 8, 10, 1988.

Merton, R. K., *Social Theory and Social Structure,* The Free Press, New York, 1968.

Rando, T. A., *Grieving: How To Go On Living When Someone You Love Dies,* D. C. Heath and Company, Lexington, Massachusetts, 1988.

Rando, T. A., *Treatment of Complicated Mourning,* Research Press, Champaign, Illinois, 1993.

Sandarupa, S., *Life and Death of the Toraja People,* CV. Tiga Taurus, Ujung, Pandang, 1984.

Stephenson, J. S., *Death, Grief, and Mourning: Individual and Social Realities,* The Free Press, New York, 1985.

Tatelbaum, J., *The Courage to Grieve,* Harper and Row, New York, 1980.

Tatelbaum, J., *You Don't Have to Suffer: A Handbook for Moving Beyond Life's Crises,* Harper & Row Publishers, New York, 1989.

The Random House Dictionary of the English Language (2nd Edition), Unabridged, Random House, New York, 1987.

Worden, J. W., *Grief Counseling and Grief Therapy,* Springer Publishing Company, New York, 1991.

RESOURCES FOR
BEREAVED PERSONS

This list of resources is by no means an exhaustive list. Each, however, has been checked by phone or letter and found to be reliable and helpful.

UNITED STATES

The Compassionate Friends, Inc.
P.O. Box 3696
Oak Brook, IL 60522
(708) 990-0010
9 A.M. to 4 P.M. CST, Monday through Friday

Extensive publications and videos on different aspects of grief for bereaved parents and siblings. Local chapters throughout the United States. Will refer caller to nearest chapter representative.

MADD (Mothers Against Drunk Driving)
511 E. John Carpenter Freeway, Suite 700
Irving, TX 75062-8187
(214) 744-MADD
1-800-GET MADD
8 A.M. to 5 P.M. CST, Monday through Friday
Twenty-four-hour answering service

Crisis intervention, emotional support, court related support, referral to local chapters for victim families; brochures, books, video tapes.

National AIDS Hotline
Twenty-four-hour hotline, 1-800-342-2437
Spanish 1-800-344-7432, 8 A.M. to 2 A.M. CST, seven days a week
TTY 1-800-243-7889, 10 A.M. to 10 PM. CST, Monday through Friday

Provides information, counseling, referrals to support groups for families, friends, and partners in local areas.

National Organization for Victim Assistance
1757 Park Road N.W.
Washington, D.C. 20010
(202) 232-6682
Twenty-four-hour hotline

Offers short-term counseling, information, referral to programs in local areas.

Parents of Murdered Children
100 East 8th Street, B-41
Cincinnati, OH 45202
(513) 721-LOVE
8 A.M. to 4 P.M. EST, Monday through Friday

Provides information, educational materials, and the telephone number of the nearest contact person.

Pregnancy and Infant Loss Center
1421 East Wayzata Boulevard #30
Wayzata, MN 55391
(612) 473-9372
9 A.M. to 4 P.M. CST, Monday through Friday

Nonprofit organization established in 1983. Provides support, resources, and education on miscarriage, stillbirth, and infant death. Publishes a quarterly newsletter, *Loving Arms*. Books, cards, and items for memory books/boxes; referral to support groups throughout the United States.

SHARE
(Source of Help in Airing and Resolving Experiences)
St. Joseph Health Center
Attention National SHARE Office
300 First Capitol Drive
St. Charles, MO 63301
(314) 947-6164
9 A.M. to 5 P.M. CST, Monday through Friday

Support, resources, counseling for bereaved parents (especially infant loss through perinatal death, newborn, neonatal, stillbirth, miscarriage); referral to local chapters.

SIDS (Sudden Infant Death Syndrome) Alliance
1314 Bedford, Suite 210
Baltimore, MD 21208
1-800-221-SIDS
Office is open from 9 A.M. to 5 P.M. EST, Monday through Friday
Twenty-four-hour emergency hotline (answering service)

Offers services to families with Sudden Infant Death Syndrome; affiliates (chapters) throughout the United States; education and information; telephone/address of nearest affiliate (chapter).

The Doughy Center
P.O. Box 86852
Portland, OR 97286
(503) 775-5683
9 A.M. to 5 P.M. PST, Monday through Friday

General information on children and grief, materials and video tapes; national training for persons interested in starting support groups for grieving children.

Theos (They Help Each Other Spiritually)
322 Boulevard of the Allies, Suite 105
Pittsburgh, PA 15222
(412) 471-7779
9:30 A.M. to 4 P.M. EST, Monday through Thursday.
Twenty-four-hour answering service

Self help programs for widows and widowers; chapters throughout the United States.

Widowed Persons Service
American Association of Retired Persons
601 E. Street N.W.
Washington, D.C. 20049
(202) 434-2260
8 A.M. to 5 P.M. EST, Monday through Friday

Referral to nearest outreach program in which trained widowed
volunteers offer support to newly widowed persons of all ages. If
no program near, will send printed material.

CANADA

Bereaved Families of Ontario
214 Merton Street, Suite 204
Toronto, Ontario, Canada M4S 1A6
(416) 440-0290
Staffed from 8:30 A.M. to 4:30 P.M. EST, Monday through Friday.

Provides written material, seminars, and support groups for
parents whose children have died and for children, adolescents,
and young adults who have lost a parent or sibling. Referrals are
made to the nearest chapter (17 chapters in Ontario) as well as
information on resources in other provinces.

The Compassionate Friends of Canada
685 William Avenue
Winnipeg, Manitoba, Canada R3E 0Z2
(204) 787-4896 / FAX: (204) 475-9527

There is a Drop In Centre on Mondays and staff is available
Thursday evenings. Messages are retrieved on a daily basis and
answered immediately. Provides a telephone friend, packet of
materials for bereaved parents, siblings, friends, co-workers, and
professionals. Offers a newsletter. There are approximately
seventy-five chapters across Canada and forty to fifty contacts in
areas with no chapter.

MADD Canada
6507C Mississauga Road
Mississauga, Ontario, Canada L5N 1A6
(905) 813-6233, EST (local Toronto calling area)
1 (800) 665-MADD, EST (toll-free Canada wide)
Office Hours: 9 A.M. to 5 P.M. (staffed)

Local chapters vary in levels of service. National Office provides information and referral services, literature, telephone victim support, victim advocate training, and Candlelight Vigil.

UNITED KINGDOM

The Compassionate Friends
53 North Street
Bristol, England BS3 1EN
(Administration) 0117 966 5202
(Helpline) 0117 953 9639

The Helpline is manned during weekdays from 9:30 A.M. to 5 P.M. For other hours, a message may be left on the answering machine or an alternative number to call is given.

Cruse-Bereavement Care
Cruse House, 126 Sheen Road
Richmond, Surrey, United Kingdom TW9 1UR
0181-940-4818
FAX: 0181 940 7638
Cruse Bereavement Line: 0181 332 7227

The numbers listed above are answered 9:30 A.M. to 5 P.M., Monday through Friday. Purports to be the largest bereavement counseling organization of its type in the world with nearly 200 branches throughout the United Kingdom. Offers counseling support groups and information on practical matters to bereaved people through the branches and the telephone Bereavement Line.

AUSTRALIA

The Compassionate Friends (Inc.)
79 Stirling Street
Perth, Western Australia 6000
Drop In Centre (09) 227 5698

Centre Hours: usually Mondays to Thursdays 10 A.M. to 3 P.M., GMT. Answering machine with emergency number at other times. Provides information on grief, healing and related issues, support meetings, memorial services, and occasional seminars.

SUGGESTED READINGS/VIDEOS

There are many books and videos on grief and grief-related issues. The following, some old, some new, are ones I recommend or have been recommended to me by a bereaved person or persons.

GENERAL

Bozarth-Campbell, *Alla, Life is Goodbye, Life is Hello: Grieving Well Through All Kinds of Loss,* CompCare Publications, 1982.

Colgrove, Melba, Harold H. Bloomfield, and Peter McWilliams, *How To Survive the Loss of a Love,* Prelude Press, 1991.

Deits, Bob, *Life After Loss: A Personal Guide to Dealing with Death, Divorce, Job Change and Relocation,* Fisher Books, 1992.

Grollman, Earl A., *Living When a Loved One Has Died,* Beacon Press, 1977.

Grollman, Earl A., *Time Remembered: A Journal for Survivors,* Beacon Press, 1987.

James, John W. and Frank Cherry, *The Grief Recovery Handbook: A Step-by-Step Program for Moving Beyond Loss,* Harper & Row, Publishers, 1988.

Kushner, Harold S., *When Bad Things Happen to Good People,* Avon Books, 1981.

Levang, Elizabeth and Sherokee Ilse, *Remembering with Love: Messages of Hope for the First Year of Grieving and Beyond,* Deaconess Press, 1992.

Manning, Doug, *Don't Take My Grief Away,* HarperCollins Publishers, 1984.

Menten, Ted, *Gentle Closings: How To Say Goodbye to Someone You Love,* Running Press, 1991.

Miller, James E., *What Will Help Me?/How Can I Help?* Willowgreen Publishing, 1994.

Moffat, Mary Jane (ed.), *In the Midst of Winter: Selections from the Literature of Mourning,* Vintage, 1982.

Neeld, Elizabeth Harper, *Seven Choices: Taking the Steps to New Life After Losing Someone You Love,* Clarkson N. Potter, Inc., 1990.

Price, Eugenia, *Getting Through the Night: Finding Your Way After the Loss of a Loved One,* Ballantine Books, 1982.

Rando, Therese A., *Grieving: How To Go On Living When Someone You Love Dies,* Lexington Books, 1988.

Rupp, Joyce, *Praying Our Goodbyes,* Ave Maria Press, 1988.

Schoeneck, Therese S., *Hope for the Bereaved: Understanding, Coping and Growing Through Grief,* Hope for the Bereaved, Inc., 1991.

Sims, Darcie D., *Why Are the Casseroles Always Tuna? A Loving Look at the Lighter Side of Grief,* Big A & Company, 1992.

Tatelbaum, Judy, *The Courage to Grieve: Creative Living, Recovery, and Growth Through Grief,* Harper and Row, 1980.

Tatelbaum, Judy, *You Don't have to Suffer: A Handbook for Moving Beyond Life's Crises,* Harper and Row, 1989.

Westberg, Granger E., *Good Grief,* Fortress Press, 1971.

YOUR HUSBAND OR WIFE DIED

Caine, Lynn, *Being a Widow,* William Morrow and Company, Inc., 1988.

Curry, Cathleen L., *When Your Spouse Dies: A Concise and Practical Source of Help and Advice,* Ave Maria Press, 1990.

Ericsson, Stephanie, *Companion Through Darkness: Inner Dialogues On Grief,* HarperPerenial, 1988.

Lewis, C. S., *A Grief Observed,* The Seabury Press, Inc., 1974.

YOUR CHILD DIED

Bolton, Iris, *My Son . . . My Son . . . A Guide to Healing After Death, Loss, or Suicide,* Bolton Press, 1983.

Heavlin, Marilyn Willett, *Roses in December,* Here's Life Publishers, Inc., 1986.

Schiff, Harriet Sarnoff, *The Bereaved Parent,* Penguin Books, 1977.

MISCARRIAGES, STILLBIRTHS, INFANT DEATHS

Ilse, Sherokee and Linda Hammer Burns, *Miscarriage: A Shattered Dream,* Wintergreen Press, 1985.

Ilse, Sherokee, *Empty Arms: Coping with Miscarriage, Stillbirth and Infant Death,* Wintergreen Press, 1990.

Ilse, Sherokee, *Precious Lives, Painful Choices,* Wintergreen Press, 1993.

Limbo, Rana K. and Sara Rich Wheeler, *When A Baby Dies: A Handbook for Healing and Helping,* Resolve Through Sharing (RTS) Bereavement Services, 1986.

RESOURCES FOR
CHILDREN AND YOUNG ADULTS

Books

Buscaglia, Leo, *The Fall of Freddie the Leaf,* Charles B. Slack, Inc., 1982.

de Paola, Tomie, *Nana Upstairs and Nana Downstairs,* Puffin Books, 1978.

Gravelle, Karen and Charles Haskins, *Teenagers Face to Face with Bereavement,* Julian Messner, 1989.

Krementz, Jill, *How It Feels When a Parent Dies,* Peter Smith, 1993.

LeShan, Eda, *Learning To Say Good-Bye When a Child's Parent Dies,* Avon Books, 1988.

O'Toole, Donna, *Aarvy Aardvark Finds Hope: A Read Aloud Story for People of All Ages,* Celo Press, 1988.

Sims, Alicia M, *Am I Still a Sister?* Big A and Company, 1986.

Traisman, Enid Samuel, *Fire in My Heart—Ice in My Veins: A Journey for Teenager Experiencing a Loss,* Centering Corporation, 1992.

Workbooks

Bisignano, Judith, *Living With Death: Journal Activities for Personal Growth,* (Grades 5-9+), Good Apple, 1991.

Boulden, Jim, *Saying Goodbye Activity Book,* Jim Boulden, P.O. Box 9358, Santa Rosa, CA 95405, 1989.

Cera, Mary Jane, *Living With Death: Activities to Help Children Cope with Difficult Situations* (Grades 1-4), Good Apple, 1991.

Heegaard, Marge Eaton, *When Someone Very Special Dies: Children Can Learn to Cope with Death,* Woodland Press, 1988.

Van-Si, Lauris and Lynn Powers, *Helping Children Heal From Loss: A Keepsake Book of Special Memories,* Continuing Education Press, Portland State University, 1944.

Helping Children

Doka, Kenneth J. (ed.), *Children Mourning: Mourning Children,* Hospice Foundation of America, 1995.

Gaffney, Donna A., *The Seasons of Grief: Helping Your Children Grow Through Loss,* New American Library, 1988.

Fitzgerald, Helen, *The Grieving Child: A Parent's Guide,* Simon and Schuster, 1992.

Grollman, Earl A., *Talking About Death: A Dialogue Between Parent and Child,* Beacon Press, 1990.

LaTour, Kathy, *For Those Who Live: Helping Children Cope with the Death of a Brother or Sister,* Centering Corporation, P.O. Box 3367, Omaha, NE 68103, 1983.

Mellonie, Bryan and Robert Ingpen, *Lifetimes: The Beautiful Way to Explain Death to Children,* Bantam Books, 1983.

Morgan, John D. (ed.), *The Dying and the Bereaved Teenager,* The Charles Press, 1990.

Schaeffer, Dan and Christine Lyons, *How Do We Tell the Children?* Newman Press, 1988.

Stevenson, Robert G. (ed.), *What Will We Do? Preparing a School Community to Cope with Crises,* Baywood Publishing Company, Inc., 1994.

AIDS

Donnelly, Katherine Fair, *Recovering From the Loss of a Loved One to AIDS: Help for Surviving Family, Friends, and Lovers Who Grieve,* Fawcett Columbine, 1994.

Jordon, MaryKate, *Losing Uncle Tim,* Albert Whitman & Company, 1989.

SUDDEN DEATH, SUICIDE, HOMICIDE

Hewett, John H., *After Suicide,* The Westminster Press, 1980.

Langford, Mary, *That Nothing Be Wasted: My Experience with the Suicide of My Son,* New Hope, Birmingham, Alabama, 1988.

Lord, Janice Harris, *No Time for Goodbyes,* Pathfinder Publishing, 1995.

Sandefer, Kathleen, *Mom, I'm Alright,* Kathleen Sandefer, 1990.

THOSE WHO WANT TO HELP

Donnelley, Nina Herrmann, *I Never Know What to Say,* Ballantine Books, 1987.

VIDEOS

Invincible Summer: Returning to Life After Someone You Loved Died (17 minutes). Guides the viewer through the natural progression of grief. Willowgreen Productions, 509 W. Washington Blvd., Fort Wayne, IN 46802.

A Taste of Blackberries, an annotated film for children (16 minutes). Educational Perspectives Associates, P.O. Box 213, Dekalb, IL 60115.

Healing Your Grief Wound, Part I: The Early Weeks (29 minutes); Part II: *The Latter Stages* (29 minutes). SpiritQuest, Box 144, Claremont, CA 91711.

The Courage to Grieve, The Courage to Grow: Recovering and Growing Through Grief (45 minutes). Judy Tatelbaum, P.O. Box 601, Carmel Valley, CA 93924.

This Healing Path, Bereaved Siblings Talk about Grief (35 minutes). The Compassionate Friends, Inc., P.O. Box 3696, Oak Brook, IL 60522.

Understanding Grief: Kids Helping Kids (14 minutes). Batesville Management Services, One Batesville Boulevard, Batesville, IN 47006-9989.

PERIODICALS

Bereavement: A Magazine of Hope and Healing, Bereavement Publishing, Inc., 8133 Telegraph Drive, Colorado Springs, CO 80920-7169.

Thanatos: A Realistic Journal Concerning Dying, Death & Bereavement, P.O. Box 6009, Tallahassee, FL 32314-9967.

CATALOGUE

Rainbow Connection: Handpicked Resources to Help People Grow Through Loss and Grief, 477 Hannah Branch Road, Burnsville, NC 28714.

INDEX